Anthroposophical Care for the Elderly

DO
RETURN
PLEASE

Anthroposophical Care for the Elderly

Annegret Camps
Brigitte Hagenhoff
Ada van der Star

Translated by Johannes M. Surkamp
Edited by Robin Jackson

Floris Books

First published in German as *Pflegemodell "Schöpferisch pflegen"*
by Info-3 Verlag, Frankfurt in 2006
First published in English by Floris Books in 2008
Third printing 2010

British Library CIP Data available

ISBN 978-086315-653-3

Printed in Great Britain by
Good News Digital Books

Contents

Foreword   9
Introduction   11
   Background   11
   The anthroposophical model of care   12
   The model of care in relation to the scientific environment   12
   The practical relevance of the model of care   14

PART 1
Fundamentals of the Anthroposophical Knowledge of Man

1. Fourfoldness   19
   The physical body   19
   The life body (etheric body)   19
   The soul body (astral body)   21
   The human 'I'   22
   Summary   24
What happens in sleep?   25
   Further reading   26

2. Threefoldness   27
   Body, soul, spirit   27
The functional threefoldness of the human organism   28
   Sensory-nervous system   28
   Metabolic-limb system   28
   Rhythmic system   29
Thinking, feeling and acting   30
   Further reading   31

3. Regarding the Senses   32
Bodily senses   33
   Sense of touch   33
   Sense of life   34

Sense of one's own movement	34
Sense of balance	34
Summary of the bodily senses	35
Social senses	35
Sense of smell	35
Sense of taste	35
Sense of sight	35
Sense of warmth	36
Summary of the social senses	36
Spiritual senses	36
Sense of hearing	37
Sense of language	37
Sense of thought	37
Sense of self and others	37
Summary of the spiritual senses	38
Further reading	38

PART 2
Selected Concepts from Anthroposophy Relevant to Care

4. The Human Being and the Environment	41
The physical body and its environment	41
The etheric body and its environment	42
The astral body and its environment	43
The 'I' and its environment	44
Further reading	45
5. The Biography	46
Stages in the development of the human being	46
The first twenty-one years (bodily development)	47
The second twenty-one years (soul development)	47
The third twenty-one years (spiritual development)	48
Summary overview	50
Further reading	50
6. Old Age	51
The physical body in old age	51
The life forces in old age	51
The soul life in old age	52

The individuality in old age   53
Challenging developments in the ageing process   54
Changes in configuration   55
Questions of meaning   56
Further reading   57

7. Health and Illness   59
Health   59
   Bodily well-being   59
   Social well-being   59
   Spiritual well-being   60
Disturbances in the health of body, soul and spirit   60
   Bodily illness   60
   Soul-related illness   61
   Spiritual illness   62
Illness and destiny   63
   Further reading   63

8. Repeated Earth Lives   65
Life after death   65
   The physical body after death   66
   The etheric body after death   66
   The astral body after death   66
   The 'I' after death   67
Preparation for a new incarnation   67
The path towards the earth   68
   Further reading   68

9. The concept of care   69
   Further reading   71

PART 3
**Guidelines for the Application of the Anthroposophical
   Model of Care**

10. Application of the model of care to practice   75
   Who is the 'resident'?   75
   10.1 Ability to communicate   76
   10.2 Ability to move   80

10.3 Ability to maintain vital functions of life   84
10.4 Ability to care for oneself   89
10.5 Ability to eat and drink   93
10.6 Ability to urinate and defecate   97
10.7 Ability to dress   101
10.8 Ability to rest, relax and sleep   104
10.9 Ability to occupy oneself   108
10.10 Ability to feel and conduct oneself as a man/woman   112
10.11 Ability to live untroubled in a secure and stimulating environment   115
10.12 Ability to secure and shape social relationships   119
10.13 Ability to deal with existential experiences in life   122
Characteristics of existential experiences   122
Dependency as an existential experience   123
Stages of confronting existential experiences   125
Existential experiences are experiences of the self   126

Endnotes   127
Bibliography   127

Foreword

This is the first publication available in English which integrates an anthroposophical approach with care planning. The book will be of special relevance for those working with the elderly. It will be of great value to those inspired by an anthroposophical insight into the human being and who wish to apply this in their nursing or care practice. An understanding of fourfoldness, the seven life processes and twelve senses has been fundamental to the work of curative education but is equally valid towards an understanding of ageing and illness.

For those not yet familiar with anthroposophical concepts and terminology the first two sections of this book attempt to give the reader an understanding of all aspects guiding the process of care planning as formulated in the final section.

Providing holistic care in a residential setting is a complex issue. Care tasks may be simple but their implications profound. The care planning section of the book is very detailed but provides helpful tools for creating comprehensive care plans based on the needs of body, soul and spirit. The questions posed challenge the caregiver to develop an empathetic understanding of another's needs and individuality.

Although the anthroposophical approach is integrated into a German model of nursing care this can be easily adapted for use in conjunction with a British framework for the activities of daily living.

We welcome this English translation and hope that many readers will find the book helpful and encouraging, leading them to a deepening in the quality of their care practice.

Judith Jones, Simeon Care for the Elderly, Aberdeen
Pirkko Lindholm, Simeon Care for the Elderly, Aberdeen
Barbara Plant, Milltown Community, Arbuthnott

Introduction

Background

For several decades there have been institutions for the care for the elderly based on Rudolf Steiner's anthroposophy. They have been guided by an image of the human being which considers, beyond the obvious and visible components, the soul and spiritual qualities. The aim of this anthroposophically oriented care for the elderly is to support the autonomy of the person in care, to maintain her social contacts and competences and, so far as it is needed, to accompany her on life's journey.

With the model of care presented here, not only do we want to meet the requirements of the relevant (German) authorities, as well as stating the theoretical basis on which the concept of care in the homes of the Nikodemus-Werk is built, but also extend an invitation to carers to apply the anthroposophical image of man to their daily work.

In the first instance it might be discouraging for practitioners to have to read 'all of this' and then apply it to their daily practice. However, carers who have read beyond the first few pages have noticed that they are not dealing with a complicated text but with comprehensible descriptions of situations found in practice.

The authors do not want this model of care to be seen as a programme which has to be realized point by point in order to make an institution 'anthroposophical' but simply as a practical tool that can be applied and tested.

It is part of professional care that in addition to the hands-on work there should be a system by which the practical acts of care can be differentiated, organized, executed, documented and financially accounted for.

The requirements of elderly people can be grasped in different ways. They can be expressed in an open and obvious way or can be recognized in a wide range of everyday activities. In order to plan care adequately it is necessary to determine the origin of these needs. For instance, it may be that an individual wishes to meet a particular need on her own. The task of the carer would not be to ignore such a wish but to ensure that the person concerned can cope in as independent a manner as possible.

The anthroposophical model of care

Through the concepts it employs the anthroposophical model of care presents an image of the human being which considers all of those facets which are relevant for care.

This enables the carer to look at people as a configuration of various elements: threefold and fourfold structures; their relationship to the environment through the senses, and the psychological development throughout their lives revealed in their biographies. Beyond this, the human being can be looked upon as a transcendental being, originating in a spiritual world and returning to it again (dying and life after death).

These concepts, which can be understood by themselves, can also build on one another. They supplement each other and contribute to understanding people and recognizing developments, even situations, which are not part of life-activities. Apart from this, they help individual carers develop their personalities in their work and support groups of carers in collaborating and communicating within a team.

Just as anthroposophy does not see itself as an alternative to other sciences, so too this model of care should be seen as an extension to other care models (see Part 3).

Whilst most models are linked to a theory that has a sound basis in scientific knowledge, the scientific foundation for the anthroposophical model has yet to be demonstrated.

The model of care in relation to the scientific environment

Models serve the purpose of simplifying reality. They are images of an observed or anticipated reality. They are meant to help explain and simplify the understanding of connections and actions.

First of all, models can be subdivided into two categories, namely *theoretical* and *empirical* models which can be created *before* or *after* the development of the theories.

> Models designed *before* the development of theories explore what has to be answered by a theory.

> Models designed *after* the development of theories help to give an overview of different theories and illustrate how different concepts are linked in order to make them understandable to the user.

The case presented here is an empirical model. We consciously chose the practical approach (*before* the formulation of a theory) and let our model arise out of more than twenty years of practical experience in the care of, and training for, the elderly.

This model is highly applicable to everyday care. It helps carers discern the phenomena deriving from this anthroposophical image of man, to recognize them in the work context and to put that in words. It is a tool which serves the purpose of creating order in one's thoughts and to set priorities. Not least, it will also make possible the description of service performance and present it in a context which does justice to the elderly in their total situation.

A.I. Meleis has presented a rough outline of these various models according to the focus of their content.[1] She differentiates:

- Models according to need (what do the carers do?)
- Models of interaction (how do the carers contribute?)
- Models determined by the result of caring (why and with what
    aim is care applied?)

Following this categorization, the model presented here is an according-to-need model. It derives from the fundamental image of man and the corresponding understanding of the nature of care. For that reason, it is not a model solely determined as a result of experience in caring for the elderly. The object, with respect to the care for the elderly, is to enhance and maintain their quality of life. The aims for this work derive from the needs of the residents and this can only be achieved through interaction with the elderly.

A further approach to the understanding of this model of care is the one offered by Hilde Steppe who presents the structured model.[2] According to this model, relevant and guiding practical activities can take account of the following:

- Aims and objectives of care
- The 'handiwork' of care
- The organization of the care-service
- Psychosocial and communicative elements
- Conditions in the work realm

These five categories are based on theoretical statements relating to:

- Image of man
- Health
- Environment
- Relationships
- Definitions of care

These include discoveries in other disciplines. In our case, these are discoveries which have been gained from an anthroposophical concept of science as the conclusions drawn from it derive from the writings of and lectures by Rudolf Steiner. Many phenomena relevant to care are described in detail in the anthroposophical supporting literature. References to these are given in the various sections.

The practical relevance of the model of care

The third part of the book will show how the anthroposophical model of care can be applied to actual care plans. The system devised by Monika Krohwinkel is provided as an example, as this is the system currently most in use. The questions formulated will help provide a checklist based on an anthroposophically image of the human being. This model of care will help inspecting authorities to recognize the specifically anthroposophical elements which inform our care institutions.

To the question of integrating this model of care in existing arrangements (for instance, mission statements; care standards; and existing documentary systems), the following illustration can be given:

> With the concepts involved in this model of care, we are dealing with basic concepts relating to the anthroposophical science of Man which are relevant to care. At this level we will be able to arrive at a common understanding through the use of objective concepts.

> At the heart of any institution there are particular ways for these to find expression. The model of care proposed needs to be developed in a way that relates to an institution's own unique circumstances.

In the guidelines or 'care standards' section, there are ways in which this model can be applied. They correspond to the range of provisions found in most care institutions. Whilst these guidelines are transferable, they have to be in harmony with the nature of the everyday work in that institution.

PART 1

Fundamentals of the Anthroposophical Knowledge of the Human Being

1. Fourfoldness

Four principles are described which are at work in every human being. All phenomena in the human being are contained in these four principles. These are: the material body (physical body), the biological processes (life processes or etheric body), the psychic parts (soul or astral-body) and the personality (self or 'I'). In every human being these four interact. The different ways in which these four principles interact give rise to the uniqueness of the individual person.

The physical body

This concept refers to what can be perceived by the senses, what can be weighed and measured.

- Weighing — relates to gravity
- Counting — relates to quantities of matter
- Measuring — relates to the expansion in physical space

All parts of the physical body can be measured. The human being is also part of the mineral world and is subject to its laws. Human beings consist physically of the same material as the *earth*. The physical body is the outer, visible form of the human being. In anatomy, this body is carefully examined and described. The care of the physical body is dependent on its being kept in order, that impurities are removed and defects put right, that the laws and knowledge relating to spatial situations and gravitational forces are recognized and applied.

The life body (etheric body)

The life body is active in the physical body of a plant, an animal and a human being which brings about life. This is manifest in seven processes:

- breathing
- warming
- nourishing
- secreting

- maintaining
- growing
- reproducing*

These seven processes of the life body are closely interrelated and are in a state of delicate balance. Not only do they complement each other quantitatively but also qualitatively, as in the sequence presented here.

The life body functions through the medium of the *element of water.* It takes hold of the physical body through its liquid (watery) component. All fluids in the human being can be bearers of life. However excreted liquids no longer carry any life. Excretion of 'dead' water and 'dead' matter leads to the removal of substances from the body (for instance, urine, sweat, sputum, pus). Accumulations of 'dead' water are found in the body (for instance, urine in the bladder). Other 'dead' waters do not have allocated places in the body; they may look for a place and create 'disturbances' (for instance, oedemas, abscesses).

The life body carries the principle of life in a sevenfold way: a principle that was already known in ancient cultures under the name of' 'etheric body.'

The life body, as such, is not visible to the eye. It is recognizable only by the effects of the seven life processes and by noticing their changes. To this end, observations are necessary over a period of time of vital functions, biological processes and rhythms. For this reason, the life body can also be called the 'time body.' The attention to rhythm, as a therapeutic factor, is very important in caring.

---

* These seven life processes can be seen concretely, for instance, in taking nourishment:

Breathing: Our need is for regular nourishment. The breathing principle shows itself in the binding and dissolution with the outside world.

Warming: Taking in nourishment produces warmth. The right warmth enables us to interact with the world.

Nourishing: Taking in nourishment enables us to extract energy and strength. The world begins to have meaning.

Secreting: The organism secretes what it does not need. The secretion principle can be seen as the ability to distinguish essential from non-essential.

Maintaining: Taking in nourishment maintains the body in its form and configuration.

Growing: If the previous five processes are harmonious, growth can take place. The growing principles can be seen as integrating new experiences.

Reproducing: All the above processes together form the basis that the body can bring forth a new human being. The reproducing principle can be seen as the ability to take in the existing, transform it, and set it into a new form.

The life processes form the realm in which most of our activity as carers takes place. We offer support, encouragement, stimulation for the maintenance and regeneration of the life processes.

In the practice of care, this means enhancing, supporting and stimulating the vital processes through nourishment and washing and external practices such as rhythmical application of ointments or oil.

The soul body (astral body)

In describing the astral body the soul level is addressed. In the soul life all sensations and movements have their home. Sensations arise on the basis of sensory perceptions and through them our sympathies and antipathies are expressed. In sympathy, one is attracted to something or one wants to unite with an object or fact which arouses sympathetic feelings. Feelings of antipathy are caused when one is repelled by something. Between attraction and repulsion, movement comes about. This has its home in the astral body.

Feelings are especially expressed in breathing. In the care of coma patients this phenomenon can be used to establish communication with the patient. If you pay careful attention to a patient's breathing — often aided by instruments that register the intensity of breathing — carers can infer from that pattern a patient's agreement (sympathy) or disagreement (antipathy).

The interplay of the depth and rhythm of breathing signifies a kind of soul language (for instance, laughing, sighing, groaning, sobbing). As the physical body is manifest in the element of earth and the life-processes show themselves active in the element of water, the expression of the soul presents itself chiefly in the *element of air.* When air and water meet, the soul life influences the life processes right into the metabolic processes. The life processes, modified by the soul, which penetrate the physical body, leave their traces visible in mime and gesture, and also in the way a person moves. In the course of time, the mime is inscribed into the physical body and during the course of life a lasting physiognomy comes about.

In this way the soul, the astral body, finds a threefold expression in the human body: firstly, directly in breathing (rhythmic system); secondly, in the metabolism and movement (metabolic-limb system); and thirdly, in the physiognomy (sensory nervous system), (see Chapter 2, Threefoldness).

All living creatures, breathing through the lung, have an astral body. Rhythmically they draw in breath into the lungs and exhale again. In the up and down of breathing, the soul life links with and loosens itself from the lower parts of the human being. In the blood a mixture of soul life and life processes comes about.

Animals and humans have such a respiratory system. Soul sensations can be studied perfectly in the movements of animals. The study of body language in animals is the basis for an understanding of animals and ways of communicating with them (for instance, trainer; horse whisperer; tamer). Every animal expresses its soul-language through specific movement patterns. We can recognize and study this language. The body language of animals differs from that of humans inasmuch as it is almost entirely limited to the movements of the whole body (gesture). Only human beings can show strongly articulated and changing facial expressions.

Animals remain in their soul-life which is directly related to their environment. With their soul they melt into their surroundings and react directly to any changes and events which may occur. Human beings in contrast avail themselves of a higher principle, a fourth member of their being, the self, the ability to refer to oneself as 'I.'*

By creating the environment, by caring for and stimulating the senses through spatial architecture, colours, aromas and sounds, the sensory experiences can be beneficially affected. This discussion is expanded in Chapters 3 (Regarding the Senses), 4 (The Human Being and the Environment), and 9 (The Concept of Care).

The human 'I'

The 'I,' or self, seen from an evolutionary point of view, is the youngest part. It only works in human beings but not in a continuous or uniform manner. The animal does not have an self; its consciousness only reaches the level of sensation. As the 'I' is of a purely spiritual nature, it is difficult to describe it. It withdraws and hides from any

---

* In the realm of movement, the higher principle, the 'I,' shows itself in the human ability to create new forms of movement (for instance, dance, sport, kinesthetics). The 'I' appears between feeling and expression, and modifies the movement. While gesture is an immediate expression of feeling, in our human facial movement the feelings are modified by our thinking (expressing, for instance, wonder, doubt, humour).

materialistic approach. It is the basis for our bright day-consciousness. The 'I' can perceive clearly and consciously stirrings of the soul and can modify them by reflecting on them.

As the life forces work in the element of water and the soul forces of the astral body work in the element of air, the 'I' works in the *element of warmth*. In order to be fully effective in the body, the 'I' needs a body temperature of 36.5 to 37.5°C (97.7–99.5°F). Enthusiasm, which produces warmth, is an expression of strong activity of the self.

In order to use the 'I,' the human being needs the ability to think, which is only possible with a wakeful consciousness.

In order to unfold the 'I,' the human being needs thought based dialogue with other human beings and needs to experience the world surrounding him. It is also necessary to be self reflective, to think, evaluate, test, choose, decide and carry responsibility.

The 'I' is the 'master in his house,' the 'charioteer' who holds the reins in his hand. The 'I' is not subject to sympathies and antipathies. One does not wander half asleep from sense impression to sense impression but choices are made. From impressions and experiences, we create our own biography as our own history.

It is the growing self-awareness of the 'I' that we understand as the 'development of individuality' and which is the basis of our own freedom.

In summary, it can be said that because human beings have an 'I':
• we have an individuality
• we have a consciousness of ourselves
• we have a wakeful consciousness
• we can distinguish between thoughts and can choose to de-
    velop them further
• we carry responsibility.

The fourfoldness in its completeness can only be found in the human being because only the human being can develop an 'I.' The description of astral body and 'I' addresses the higher parts of the human being.

Summary

Principle	physical body	life body	soul body	I (self)
Characteristics	space, weight, matter	breathing, warming, nourishing, secreting, maintaining, growing, reproducing	sensations, sympathy, antipathy, own movement	autonomy, thinking, responsibility, decisions
Nature	mineral kingdom	plant kingdom	animal kingdom	human kingdom
Consciousness	no consciousness	sleeping consciousness	dreaming consciousness	waking consciousness
Element	earth (solid)	water	air	fire (warmth)
Visibility	visible	invisible, but effects seen in course of time	invisible, but effects seen in form and movement	invisible, but effects seen in biography of individual development
Relevance for care	Keeping order	Maintaining vital functions and biological processes	Recognize soul quality in social meeting. Stimulate by creating the environment	Valuing individuality through meeting as partners. Giving space for individual development

What happens in sleep?

During the day the human being uses part of his life forces in order to maintain his consciousness. Sensory activity and thinking use up energy which is supplied by the etheric body. This energy is no longer available for the life processes. All daily activities — movement, work and play — as well as ideas and feelings, require energy.

In consequence the physical body suffers exhaustion. Therefore the human being feels used up and tired. Spiritually he feels rich in impressions. His brain is 'full' with sense impressions of daily happenings.

In sleep the astral body and the 'I' free themselves from the confinement of the physical body. They expand into their original sphere (see Chapter 4, The Human Being and the Environment). Remaining behind in bed is the physical body, now fully penetrated by the energy of the life body. This can now, unhindered by the senses' impressions, perform its sevenfold work through the life processes — restoring the strength of the human being through sleep.

The astral body 'discharges' the day's impressions into the planetary world (the processing of soul impressions) and can then 'fill up' anew with planetary forces.

This expansion of the astral body occurs about four times during the night. In the intervals, the phase of rapid eye movement (REM-phases), the astral body contracts in the direction of the physical body. During the REM-phases, the astral body can give structural impulses to the etheric body: the etheric body receives orders to restore the physical body. Everything that during the day has been damaged or over-strained (for instance by exhaustion, shock, a heavy meal, etc.) is again restored to its original state and replenished.

In the REM-phase, dreams usually develop which often reflect the interrelationship between the astral body and life body. The REM-phases are recognizable by the rapid eye movements behind the closed eyelids. If a person is frequently woken during the REM-phases, then the fresh impulses for the etheric body are curtailed, which in the long run can cause severe health damage at the physical and psychological level.

The 'I' dwells during sleep in the realm of the fixed stars and there meets the higher self, that part which has (not yet) fully incarnated into earthly life and therefore remains untouched by events on earth. The 'everyday I' encounters the higher self. Decisions and judgements are reviewed and possibly put right in relation to this archetypal image.

Therefore it can be that a person has made a decision in the evening and wakes in the morning with the sure feeling that this decision has to be revised.

A further aspect of the nightly journey is the fact that the 'I' of all human beings asleep during the same time are together in the sphere of the fixed stars without being coloured by the astral forces. These pure I-encounters can lead to changes in the relationship between people during the waking periods on earth. In this context a possible explanation may be advanced for the phenomenon of 'estrangement' encountered by a carer on continuous night duty when sleeping and waking periods have been reversed.

People have different needs for sleep. In general it can be said that the total time of sleep corresponds to a third of a lifetime. Babies need the most sleep; they also have the longest REM-phases. As they get older, as a general rule, people sleep for shorter periods of time and the REM-phases diminish in length and intensity. A good, deep sleep usually has a positive influence on the following waking period.

FURTHER READING

Borbély, Alexander, *Secrets of Sleep.*
Burkhard, Gudrun, *Taking Charge: Your Life Patterns and their Meanings.*
Camps, Annegret & Ada van der Star, *Menschenkundliche Aspekte zur Qualität in der Krankenpflege.*
Houten, Coenraad van, *Awakening the Will: Principles and Processes in Adult Learning.*
—, *Practising Destiny: Principles and Processes in Adult Learning.*
Steiner, Rudolf, *Theosophy.*
—, *Inner Reading and Inner Hearing*, lecture of Dec 19, 1914.
—, *An Outline of Esoteric Science,* Chapter 3, Sleep and Death.

2. Threefoldness

The idea of threefoldness is a basic tenet of anthroposophical thought through which an understanding of the human being and world can be gained. It is always applicable when opposites (polarities) are bridged, reconciled or mediated by a third force. Thereby three differentiated qualities appear as a totality (for instance the human being as a unity of body, soul and spirit).

Body, soul and spirit

By means of the spirit we are enabled to think, in the soul we experience feelings, and the body is our instrument to act. Just as body-soul-spirit are three and yet one, in the same way our thinking, feeling and our actions are linked together. They complement each other.

Spirit — thinking — head
Soul — feeling — heart
Body — action — hand

Body and spirit are polarities. The body is material; it is a part of earthly nature and is filled with enlivened matter. It is visible, touchable and follows the laws of physics, chemistry, biology and physiology.

In contrast to this, the spirit is invisible and therefore cannot be comprehended in a material sense. The spirit lives according to spiritual laws, which can be designated as 'higher wisdom,' 'cosmic order,' or more figuratively as 'heavenly.' No longer can physics be of use but meta-physics (*meta*, beyond) is needed to research those things which lie 'behind the visible' and which underlie them spiritually. The soul spans the bridge between heaven and earth and lives in many shades: sometimes turned more to the earthly side of life and at other times turned more to the heavenly side. In the soul both worlds meet.

Care, which in this sense is based on a holistic understanding of the human being, will always pay heed to these three elements: sometimes focusing on bodily and functional needs, sometimes on the soul component and sometimes on the spiritual part of the person in need of care.

The functional threefoldness of the human organism

Looking at the anatomical-physiological form of the body, three other differentiated qualities can be seen which form a unity. We differentiate first the polarity between the sensory-nervous system and the metabolic-limb system. Uniting and harmonizing both is the rhythmic system with heart, circulation and breathing.

Sensory-nervous system

Nerves penetrate the entire organism and have their centre in the brain. The head is the locality with the highest concentration of nerve tissue and in which most of the sensory organs are situated.

Of the three body cavities (skull, thorax, abdomen), the head is the smallest. In view of the manifoldness of functions taking place there, it is surprising how in such a small space the billions of nerve cells and passages can cope. They have little material volume, are highly specialized and sensitive and have hardly any capacity for regeneration. On a daily basis nerve cells die in the brain without being replaced. Protected by layers of skin and liquid, the brain rests motionless in the bony skull.

Nerves neither move nor swell up, even when active. Quite the opposite: any swelling or concussion constitutes a serious danger for the brain, as it disturbs the functioning of the nerves and dims or destroys consciousness.

Metabolic-limb system

The centre for the metabolic limb system is located in the cavity of the abdomen. In contrast to the nervous system, we find strong vitality and an abundance of space and round forms that swell and shrink. Constant transformation and movement is the physiological task. Metabolism means the continuous dissolving of imbibed matter and also its transformation and distribution in the organism. As a result nothing remains for long in any one place; even the bones which give the impression of permanence (remaining longest after death), are continuously involved in the metabolic process of anabolic and catabolic activity. In the limbs, the products of metabolism (sugar, protein and fat) are transformed into movement.

Rhythmic system

The thorax, situated between the sensory nerve and metabolic systems, harbours the heart and lungs as the centre of the rhythmic system. The rhythmic system bridges the polarity between metabolic system and nerves by possessing qualities common to the opposite sides and thereby balancing them. The organism would not be fit for life if these polarities confronted each other directly and there was no healthy bridging mechanism that could affect a balance between them. Complete stillness of the nervous system and continuous movement of the metabolic system find their mediator in the measured rhythm of heartbeat and breathing. Contraction of the heart muscles causes firmness for a short moment: relaxing causes the heart to swell briefly. The lungs, too, expand and contract.

The strongly pronounced quality of form in the head, which has a tendency to symmetry, contrasts with the total asymmetry of the organs of digestion. In the rhythmic system we find pair-like organs that at first sight appear symmetrical but on closer examination show marked morphological differences between right and left.

When the organism encounters the environment, all three systems show this phenomenon of polarity and balance.

If we perceive something with our senses, no matter is absorbed as a result. However much we perceive an object, touch it, feel it, taste or hear it — we always recognize forms and structures, while matter and nerves remain separate. Therefore no expression for this process is more apt than *in-formation*: a form is taken hold of, we impress ourselves with something, and we gain impressions through perception.

It is entirely different when we accept nourishment. We accept matter into ourselves, we react to it with physiological 'aggression' using both our chewing tools and muscles and the action of digestive juices so that the form and structure of what is ingested are completely obliterated. Anything that does not enter the blood through the villus is excreted (in the case of illness, it is ejected dramatically). In sensory perception, the form is accepted and matter is rejected. In the case of nourishment, matter is accepted and form rejected.

We also recognize the balancing position of breathing between sensory perception and the taking in of nourishment. Air is neither rejected nor broken down but is moved rhythmically to and fro, allowing the exchange of the gases in the organism. This process through the blood is beneficial to both realms: the nerves and the metabolism.

Thinking, feeling and acting

The sensory nervous system, rhythmic system and metabolic system form the physiological basis which enable the human being to think, feel and act. Again we meet a polarity: thinking and acting. One needs inwardness, quiet, concentration, whilst the other is an expression of activity and movement which is directed outward. Thinking requires a cool head, whilst muscular activity requires warmth.

The middle realm, feeling, has its bodily-organic correspondence in the breath and heartbeat of the rhythmic system. Just as heart and lungs are physiologically permanently changing between contraction and expansion, so feelings can swing between happiness and sorrow. One-sided thinking, which is separated from reality, is in danger of being 'icy cold.' One-sided acting can become chaotic and at worst, destructive. Only when thinking and acting mutually influence each other do they become human.

The interplay between thinking and doing is accompanied by feelings that give us the necessary intuition for the truth of thoughts and the goodness of deeds. Clear thinking on the one hand and skilful technique on the other, when joined by open sensitivity will lead to meaningful actions. A bridge is built between theory and practice.

	nerve-sense system	rhythmic system	metabolic-limb system
centre	head	thorax	abdomen, limbs
vitality	almost dead	balanced	strong vitality
form and matter	form pole, strongly formed, little material, thin, symmetrical	paired	material pole, much material, swelling forms, asymmetrical
movement	no movement, concentration	rhythmic movement	continual movement, distribution
relation to environment	perception (not material)	breathing (fine material)	nourishing and secretion
ability	thinking	feeling	acting

How does the threefoldness of the human being relate to fourfoldness? In the body, the physical body and the life body form a unity; in the soul, life and sensation are united; in the spirit, sensation and the 'I' are united.

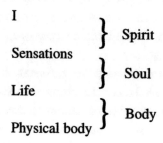

FURTHER READING

Steiner, Rudolf, *Theosophy.*
—, *An Outline of Esoteric Science.*

3. Regarding the Senses

The human being as a fourfold being is a system in its own right. In order to live on earth and communicate with one's surroundings and to develop thoughts and feelings about the world, the human being has to come into a relationship with the environment.

This contact is formed through the senses. Beyond the classical six senses (hearing, sight, touch, taste, smell and balance) the anthroposophical image of man presents six further senses by which a person receives sensory impressions of the world around. These are: the sense of life, of (one's own) movement, of warmth, of language, of thought, and of self. Accordingly, the senses can be presented in three groups:

Bodily senses: *relating to perceptions about one's own body*
• sense of touch
• sense of life
• sense of one's own movement
• sense of balance

Social senses: *relating to one's outer surroundings*
• sense of smell
• sense of taste
• sense of sight
• sense of warmth

Spiritual senses: *relating to the invisible behind the outer world*
• sense of hearing
• sense of language
• sense of thought
• sense of self

Newborn children have consciously to learn to use their senses. To begin with children learn through direct encounter with their surroundings, to which they open themselves without reserve. Only in the course of childhood and youth do they learn to consciously categorize and judge sensory experiences.

In the course of life, as ever more sensory experiences are internalized, a person can consciously gain soul-spiritual qualities through sensory experience (sublimation). For example, from bodily equilibrium the human being can achieve a balance of soul from which spiritual tranquillity can develop. We can feel that however much our soul is shaken (caught off balance), we are not blown over, for we have gained the ability to quietly take one step at a time, change what can be changed and accept what has to be accepted without getting upset.

This metamorphosis (transformation) of bodily sense perception into soul-spiritual faculties is called a sublimation of sensory activity. In the course of life the sense organs gradually degenerate so that the surroundings are no longer perceived with immediate clarity. This spiritual ability to sublimate sense impressions, once gained, enables one to deal wisely with the experiences encountered in the course of one's life. Soul-spiritual development makes a person even more human.

Human development from birth to death is due to the transformation of sensory perceptions. During the course of life there is an increasing shift towards the development of soul-spiritual faculties. Sensory activities happen on different levels:

• In the body, on the physical level, the brain serves to imprint perceptions.
• The soul is the field in which these perceptions are felt.
• The 'I' (spirit) is the authority which selects the sensations, sorts them out and makes them clear and lifts them into consciousness (processing).

For the 'I' and the soul, the physical body with the different life-processes is part of the perceived environment. In daily life, perceptions consist of a complex interplay of several senses. For instance, food 'tastes' good when it looks appetizing (sense of sight), has the right consistency (sense of touch), is the right temperature (sense of warmth), smells pleasantly (sense of smell), is well prepared (sense of taste), and is easily digestible (sense of life).

Bodily senses

Sense of touch

The sense of touch functions via the skin. We experience touch by sensing pressure and resistance. Thereby we meet the border between the 'I' and the world. We sense the heaviness of our own body.

Sublimation
Through the sense of touch we get to know the border between what is our own and what belongs to the other. The recognition of what belongs to the other demands respect. The attitude that can arise here is reverence. Curiosity is the (disrespectful) transgression of the limits.

Sense of life

The sense of life tells us whether our body is functioning harmoniously or not. When problems arise then we notice it through a headache, upset stomach, pains, sickness, and muscle cramp.

Sublimation
To experience our own pain through the sense of life forms the basis for understanding the pain experienced by others. The faculty to alleviate pain and to give comfort develops from compassion.

Sense of one's own movement

We can change the position of different parts of our body without having to look whether our legs are crossed or our head is turned to the side. The sense informing body position is the sense of our own movement. By means of this sense we generally notice movement. The organs for this sense are the cross-striped muscles.

Sublimation
Just as the perception and control of our own movements facilitate directed action, so on a higher level, we can direct our steps in life in such a way that we can turn our aims into reality.

Sense of balance

In relation to the environment we can also alter our position, for example by choosing to stand upright which is possible through the sense of balance. Through this sense we can independently change our bodily position.

Sublimation
Balance helps an individual find their own centre. If we do not want to become completely self-absorbed, we need the balance which arises

from the tension between our environment and our own centre. Only in complete equilibrium, unhindered by obstacles, does the human being experience their own centre without losing sight of the surroundings. By exercising balance, we can establish harmony between ourselves and the world. An egotist is someone who loses sight of the surrounding world. The drunkard or the enraptured person loses their own centre.

Summary of the bodily senses

The sense of touch separates a person in the first instance from the world. The senses of life and self movement provide information concerning one's own body. The sense of balance leads the person again into the world.

Social senses

Sense of smell

We receive and perceive smells through the olfactory nerves. Smells always result where a substance is in the process of disintegration. The olfactory nerve is the shortest nerve in the brain. It transmits the smell impulse directly (without synapses) to the brain. In smelling, a person has a very direct perception of the disintegrating substance.

Sublimation
Smells appear in the first instance as either pleasant or unpleasant. This evaluation tempts us to making a moral judgement of 'good' or 'bad' and may prevent further exploration of the origin of the smell. And by so doing, further development is blocked. Only by sniffing more carefully can further information be transmitted and then a qualitative indication made (for instance, wild rose, coffee). Absence of prejudice opens the door for discovering a real interest and the answers to the 'how' and 'what.'

Sense of taste

By dissolving a substance in the mouth with saliva, the sense of taste can give information about its chemical composition. Apart from the qualities of taste (for instance, sweet, sour, salty, bitter) more complex tastes can be registered (for instance, sweet milk chocolate from Lindt; Burgundy or Chianti wine).

Sublimation
In taste the chemical composition is analysed. Metaphorically speaking, taste expresses what 'fits together' (for instance, which pieces of clothing go together; which particular people to group together at a party).

Sense of sight

The eye transmits the perception of colourful surfaces. Everything else that is seen by the eye (for instance how fast a car is coming towards you) is a combination of the sense of sight and other senses as well as experience (for instance, Is the brown stain you see dried blood, chocolate, rust, or dung? Are the flowers real or made of plastic and silk?).

Sublimation
Even though some situation may present itself in a certain way, we should not jump to conclusions before looking at the situation from as many points of view as possible.

Sense of warmth

The sense of warmth informs about temperature *differences* between our body and the surrounding world. Perceptions of temperature are relative. They are always experienced in relation to something else (for instance, an outside temperature of more than 30°C/86°F will make a room temperature of 22°C/72°F feel cool).

Sublimation
The perception of warmth is a relative matter. Warm interest lies between glowing enthusiasm and cold disdain.

Summary of the social senses

The way that the four social senses relate information about the environment triggers certain feelings. As a next step, we can objectify these feelings through reflection. These feelings and thoughts initially remain in the realm of one's personal experience.

Spiritual senses

Sense of hearing

The ear receives sound waves. Besides the volume of sound qualitative criteria are also taken into account (for instance, the height and depth of tones; the warmth of a voice). Hearing involves more than just receiving sound waves.

Sublimation
The purer sound and the cleaner the air, the clearer will the tone reveal its quality. In order to develop one's perceptivity to these qualities, it is necessary to silence one's preconceptions and prejudices.

Sense of language

Beyond the quality of sound, language communicates a message beyond what is heard. Whilst language makes use of the ears, other senses are called into play if the message is to be understood. Messages can be conveyed in various ways (for instance, by gesture, symbols, hieroglyphs, or even the configuration of a group of people).

Sublimation
Language communicates a meaning beyond what is initially presented; the message needs to be decoded. The sublimation of language means accepting the outer world not as something meaningless but as something like a book from which one reads.

Sense of thought

The sense of thought is that sense which decodes the message and grasps the meaning behind the message. By so doing, it is possible to decipher, to reflect upon and grasp the significance of the communication. It is the thought that lies *behind* speech that is sought.

Sublimation
By sublimating the sense of thought, the world gains in meaning and life makes sense.

Sense of self

The sense of self can also be called the sense for the other, as it recognizes the other as a unique personality with an 'I.'

Sublimation
The recognition of the other as an independent personality, is the prerequisite for an encounter from 'I' to 'I' and through which something new can reveal itself.

FURTHER READING

Soesman, Albert, *Our Twelve Senses: Wellspring of the Soul.*

PART 2

Selected Concepts from Anthroposophy Relevant to Care

4. The Human Being and the Environment

An important aspect of care is the environment in which that care takes place. Therefore particular emphasis is placed on this aspect in models and theories of care. The surroundings in which the human being can be found are described from different points of view. Here are three essential ones:

- *natural surrounding:* This includes the earth and its climate right down to an individual's own furnished room.
- *social environment:* This comprises relatives, friends, neighbours and, more broadly, society.
- *spiritual environment:* This includes cultural elements such as art, philosophy, ethics and religion.

In the model of care that is presented here, the environment is described from an anthroposophical understanding of the world. A basic prerequisite for understanding anthroposophy is an acceptance of the hypothesis that everything has its origin in the spirit. In anthroposophically oriented care it is necessary to make this spiritual quality understandable, meaningful and recognizable in daily care situations.

The environment of the human being is described from the perspective of fourfoldness which is described in an earlier section. Thus we speak about the contribution that certain forces make which are available to human beings during their lifetime. This will now be explained.

The physical body and its environment

The physical body is the material body of the human being, which we can see, bump into, touch and take hold of. The physical body consists of mineral matter taken from the environment and ingested through nutrition. These substances are arranged in such a way that they form the human *Gestalt.* The particular manner in which these substances are arranged allows us to speak of a 'body.' If a physician wants to know how much iron is contained in the blood, he is interested in one particular substance. But only the totality of all substances, in their specific composition, makes up a **physical body.**

The physical body obeys the laws of the physical world. It is subject to the laws of gravity and occupies space. Where a physical body is, there can be no other matter. Yet this body is also separate from the physical world and is not entirely subjected to its laws. It does not dissolve in rain, or freeze in frost or necessarily tumble over on a sloping plane. During life the physical body maintains its existence as separate from the earth. Only with death does it stop being a 'body' and becomes once again completely at one with the mineral world. This physical body, with which we identify ourselves throughout our life, is actually 'on loan' from the physical earth.

The etheric body and its environment

The life forces or etheric forces express themselves in the fluid element. It is not the water itself but the energy generated by the sun which causes the processes that 'take hold' of the water and allow the life processes to come about (that is, breathing, warming, nourishing, secreting, maintaining, growing and reproducing). These delicate chemical processes repeatedly bring about different conditions of the physical matter. Water flows, seeps, streams, pulsates and springs forth in physical substances and permeates the body with the power of life. These phenomena permeate everything alive on earth whether they are plants, animals or human beings. Even the earth itself is permeated by living water.

In the etheric realm, in the life processes, all people are linked with each other and with all living things. Any disturbance affects human beings sooner or later. This is evident when, in a team of carers, one member falls ill. If a team wants to achieve the same result as on the previous day, it has to make up for the absentee's work. For the staff members this might have consequences that extend into their private lives. Also the staff member who is ill may require support or medical attention in order to recover.

What is described here on a small scale has significance for the whole of the earth. Abundance and prosperity for one part of mankind results in hunger and want for the other. Dramatic impacts on natural life patterns like monocultures, exploitation, deforestation, river diversions can cause a breakdown in the ecological balance of the whole earth. All human beings during their life on earth are called upon to take care not only of their own physical body and personal health but also the health of the whole earth (global health) because their life forces are united with the whole earth.

Like the physical body, the etheric body is only 'on loan' from the etheric forces of the earth. Every living creature gives up its life configuration (etheric body) on death and returns it to the general etheric forces of the earth.

The astral body and its environment

In the same way that the physical body belongs to the material earth and the etheric body to the etheric forces of the earth, so too the astral body has a homeland from which its forces are lent. The astral body belongs to the astral world.

The working of the planets determines the realm of the astral forces: Mercury and Venus which are closer to the sun than the earth; Mars, Jupiter, Saturn, Uranus and Neptune which are more distant from the sun than the earth. They do not themselves constitute the astral world; they delineate it. They show in their different orbits, distances and relationships, how the astral forces are active.

The planets move strictly according to the laws of the celestial world. In their orbits and various conjunctions they form mathematically exact relationships. Each planet follows its own course with its own speed. Together they form certain aspects. From each individual planet certain forces emanate that give to human beings their specific body configuration and to each organ its special form, structure and task.

Heart, liver, kidneys etc. show in their form and function the physical expression of the planetary forces with which they are permeated. For example, the gall bladder is especially related to Mars forces. When these forces are fully active it contracts strongly and the bitter juice of the gall attacks the fat in our food. When applied to the qualities of the soul, these forces provide the means to tackle problematic situations with courage.

This differs from the Venus forces that give to human beings the capacity to please others and an artistic sense for composition. Colours, sounds and tones are expressions of planetary influences. They are all based on mathematical structures that can be traced back to different combinations of planetary forces. The visible, audible world, the world experienced through the senses expresses the manifoldness and effectiveness of the astral world. Specific soul qualities are influenced by the world of the planets.

In animals these faculties are more pronounced. Every species of animals expresses specific planetary forces (for instance, the faithfulness of a dog; the courage of a lion; the gracefulness of a deer). The human being unites in his astral body many such characteristics. Every human being carries within themselves their own astral dominance. This is evident in the shape of the body and becomes even more recognizable when one considers the diversity of human souls.

It is in the nature of human souls to form communities that can be based on work or wider family relationships. In this web of contacts, astral forces are at work which become evident in many different dispositions:

- Mars force — courageous or quarrelsome
- Venus force — constructive, reconciliatory
- Mercury force — quick, cheerful, flexible
- Jupiter force — conservative, holding on

Whenever one generalizes about human behaviour, one is speaking about certain astral configurations. Operant conditioning (behaviour modification) addresses the astral body irrespective of whether it is directed to an animal or a human being. However the human being is able to control his behaviour through his own 'I' for only the 'I' can intentionally regulate and work upon the soul forces either promoting or holding them back.

The 'I' and its environment

The 'I' has its home in the world of the fixed stars characterized by the zodiac with its twelve star-signs. Other cultures, like the Chinese, are familiar with the zodiac but in different forms. The fixed stars retain their positions relative to each other. According to the season and therefore depending on the relation of the earth to the sun, they are visible at different times of night, or not visible during the day. Seen from the earth the vernal equinox moves through the zodiac in approximately 26,000 years. This means it takes about 2,150 years for the equinox to pass through one sign of the zodiac. At present the sun is moving through the sign of Pisces and will soon arrive in Aquarius.

Each individual lives in the here-and-now of his culture and takes on responsibility for his life within that culture. On earth, as independent personalities, we are able to make our own decisions. To carry responsibility for this is an activity of the 'I.' The 'I' can make a choice which may go against our own inclination or even in spite of our own feelings. The 'I' is that part of the human being which safeguards the continuity from one incarnation to the next. It is the core of the human being and sets him apart from the animals.

In the time between death and rebirth, as well as during the night, the 'I' dwells in the world of the fixed stars. There it finds its orientation and direction and there its aim and development are judged. The 'I' is the youngest member of the human being. It does not yet fully reveal itself in earthly incarnation. A part of the 'I' remains during earthly life in its fixed-star-homeland (the higher 'I') that is part of its 'environment.'

It is one of the goals of humanity to become aware of this higher 'I' and to make it ever more real on earth. This requires the possibility to make mistakes. When mistakes, not just one's own, are made they can be seen as learning opportunities which lead to further development.

From what is described here, it is clear that the 'I' differs greatly from the other parts of our being. The 'I,' unlike these other parts, is not 'on loan' to us but is the centre and pivotal point in each human being. Each 'I' is a world of its own. When in a state of wakeful I-consciousness, the human being can create new spheres of reality (for instance, science, art, philosophy and religion) which are not part of the given environment.

FURTHER READING

Steiner, Rudolf, *Theosophy*.
—, *An Outline of Esoteric Science*.

5. The Biography

A biography is more than a stringing together of life events. Each stage of life has its own quality and specific significance that is important for the gradual development of what a human being wants to become during their lifetime. Two factors determine the biography of every person:
- the 'developmental laws' according to which interaction takes place
- the events and situations which a person encounters from the outside.

Biographical development takes place in rhythms of seven-year-periods. The 'I,' the individuality, the core of the human being, holds the thread throughout the biography. In the biography, it becomes evident who a person really is.

Stages in the development of the human being

With conception the physical body is genetically determined and with birth an individual enters physically into earthly life. The other three parts (life body, soul body and 'I') permeate the physical body increasingly during the course of one's life until they fully unite.

The first twenty-one years (bodily development)

1. The first seven years: from birth to 7
The life body progressively learns to take on independently the functioning of the organs that during the embryonic development were embedded in the life forces of the mother. During the first few years of life the organism is still very tender, labile and prone to illnesses. Growth is stronger than at any other time, the body-weight doubling within only a few weeks. The organs, established before birth, now undergo a maturing process: nutrition and excretion systems learn gradually to cope with solid food. The warmth regulation becomes stabilized. The most difficult task, and at the same time the culmination of this phase, is the formation of the second teeth. School age is reached by the end of this phase.

2. The second seven years: 7 to 14

The life forces that are freed from part of their physical tasks can now stimulate the conscious forming of thoughts and the child can increasingly develop intellectual faculties. The soul body becomes more strongly integrated and establishes in puberty the precondition for a life of soul in the physical body. Bodily this is shown not only in sexual maturity but also in changes in the organs of breathing, which are closely connected to the life of feelings. In the chest the lungs have increased their volume, the face has taken on a new appearance by the maturing of the sinuses and the enlargement of the nose (the childlike snub-nose disappears). The body is still growing; strength and skill of the limbs are increasing.

3. The third seven years: 14 to 21

Once young people have fully arrived on earth emotionally, they now explore thoroughly all the heights and depths of feeling; education comes to an end and orientation towards one's own life comes to the fore. The 'I' increasingly unites with the developing and maturing human being. Towards the end of this phase, at around twenty-one years, the young adult has a fully incarnated 'I' at its disposal. The 'I,' as the youngest part of the human being, unites fully with earthly human existence. Because the three higher parts only unite step by step with the physical body, we can speak of full incarnation only from the age of twenty-one. Bodily growth, too, has come to an end. From this point, a person is considered mature and able to be self-responsible.

The second twenty-one years (soul development)

In the next twenty-one years human beings learn to develop independently, to establish their own place in life and give it shape through the 'I' by taking charge of questions of health, learning to balance and educate one's emotional life, and planning and undertaking the next steps towards self-development.

4. The fourth seven years: 21 to 28

Young adults look for their own path. They leave their parental home and 'wander' into the world. Events which take place during this phase are often the choice of profession and partner. These choices are strongly determined by feeling. This period is a development of sentient life (the *sentient soul*). The guiding questions are: 'What satisfies my feelings?' 'What touches my heart?' 'What can arouse my enthusiasm?' During this period the young person's 'I' takes hold of his feeling life and forms ideals that act as guiding stars for the future and 'better world.'

5. The fifth seven years: 28 to 35
Towards the end of the twenties this development deepens. People feel the need to take on specific responsibilities and make something of their practical life and to give shape to something. The mind is now the dominating factor. This period is a development of rational life (the *mind soul*). Important events during this phase are the founding of one's family, accepting responsibilities, committing oneself to a profession, buying a house, establishing a company, etc. The leading questions here are: What is my place? How can my contribution to the world be of use and make sense?

6. The sixth seven years: 35 to 42
The deepening becomes more intensive the more the person identifies with his tasks and responsibilities. In professional life the priorities may be the expansion of one's business or realm of work or doing better in comparison with others (competition) or making a greater profit. This second phase is rich in work, movement and events. In this phase the personality and earthly circumstances gradually come into a dialogue. It is a development of consciousness (the *consciousness soul*). This is accompanied by corresponding developments in depths of feeling, social skills and rationality. This phase of life is shaped and carried by natural gifts and temperaments as well as by education and social background.

The third twenty-one years (spiritual development)

After this first phase of maturing (approximately from the fortieth year onwards) a certain restlessness and dissatisfaction with the course of one's life can arise. This mood is often the soil from which wishes arise that give a different slant on one's own life or profession or add a new dimension to one's life. This departure from the old often goes hand in hand with separation and/or a new choice of profession (and training), particularly when it seems possible to transforms situations, when life has become 'stuck.'

Seventh seven year period: 42–49
Eighth seven year period: 49–56
Ninth seven year period: 56–63

During this period the soul body, life body and physical body become further transformed and individualized. This is evident as the life forces and soul forces no longer link up so intensively with the physical body. The outer signs are that from about forty years the first symptoms of ageing start to appear. Bodily, people no longer have the same capacities as in their thirties. The skin shows the first wrinkles, the capacity of the lungs gets smaller, and the sensory functions gradually diminish. Also the short-time memory begins to show certain deficiencies. The slow emancipation of the soul forces from the physical body becomes evident (for instance, the reduction of emotional excitability; the change of life in women with the menopause). On the other hand, those life and soul forces that are freed from activity in the physical body now reveal themselves in the ability to have a wider overview in thinking. Greater certainty arises in one's own judgement and leadership qualities can develop.

From about the 56 the personal identification with one's body changes. People engage less in physical activities now and they may be in the position to help other people to realize their ideals. They may act in a counselling capacity to others. From about 63 the inner development depends less on outer achievement. What is important now is:

• the ability to disengage from the material life (transformation of the bodily forces);
• to practise independence from one's state of health in regard to feeling well (transformation of the soul forces); and
• to turn to overarching ideas, philosophical and transcendent themes (transformation of spiritual forces).

If these transformations are successful a person can with inner composure and presence of mind develop wisdom. If this is not achieved, consciousness may focus increasingly on the degenerative symptoms of the body and accordingly more suffering is likely to be experienced. Another symptom that can occur is that the person shows less interest in earthly affairs.

The older a person becomes, the more the biography becomes individual and deviates from any general rule. Because of this a special meaning can be attributed to age and particularly old age. What counts here is to accept and recognize one's own destiny and to find the right conclusion. We therefore devote a special chapter to ageing.

Summary overview

The first twenty-one years (0–21 years: bodily development)
Physical body, etheric body (life body), astral body (soul body) and the I are 'born'; bodily maturing is completed; soul and spiritual development have started and require further development.

The second twenty-one years (21–42 years: soul-development)
The soul life stabilizes and differentiates into sentient, mental and conscious expressions; a person reaches 'mid-life.' Spiritual development has not yet reached its zenith.

The third twenty-one years (42–63 years: spiritual development)
Bodily capacities diminish and spiritual faculties can grow. Through the awareness of the finite nature of earthly life, inner qualities gain greater significance than outer success.

The later years of life
Liberation from general laws of development and the individual experience of ageing, add the final touches to one's life.

FURTHER READING

Bryant, William, *The Veiled Pulse of Time: an Introduction to Biographical Cycles and Destiny.*
Burkhard, Gudrun, *Taking Charge: Your Life Patterns and their Meanings.*
—, *Biographical Work: the Anthroposophical Basis.*
Lievegoed, Bernard, *Phases: the Spiritual Rhythms of Adult Life.*
—, *Man on the Threshold: Challenge of Inner Development.*
O'Neil, George and Gisela, *The Human Life.*
Treichler, Rudolf, *Soulways: Development, Crises and Illnesses of the Soul.*

6. Old Age

Old age, like childhood, youth and adulthood, is a phase of life in which developmental processes take place. Though the bodily forces diminish and the surroundings get more confined, it should in no way be seen as a decline. Rather it should be looked upon as a time in which differentiated processes take place and the parts of the human being undergo characteristic and varied changes. Whereas in the first half of life (as described in the previous chapter) the higher human parts connect themselves increasingly with the body (incarnation), from the middle of life, they start to loosen themselves again (excarnation). These changes are described below.

The physical body in old age

From the 'biological' middle of life (approximately age 35) the physical body increasingly becomes subjected to gravity (that is, the catabolic tendencies become stronger than the anabolic ones). It is increasingly difficult for the life forces to bring about regeneration. The physical body becomes denser and drier, loses flexibility and becomes more fragile. It is noticeable that the vital functions permeate the physical body less and less. The blood pressure rises, the metabolism is less able to cope, vessels become harder, the growth of hair is reduced and ageing symptoms become visible.

The life forces in old age

With respect to the life forces:
- breathing becomes shallower
- less warmth is produced
- some food allergies may develop
- body maintenance becomes slower (for instance, healing of wounds)
- physical changes appear (for instance, age-related patches on the skin)
- excretion becomes slacker
- growths occur (for instance, tumours)
- the reproductive faculty in women comes to an end.

When life forces become less tied to the body, they can be freed and become effective at a higher plane. An earlier freeing of the life forces occurs when the child changes teeth. From this point the life forces can be used for learning in school.

In ageing the life forces, by becoming 'free' from predominantly physical tasks, can once more be used in the service of a further development of thinking.

Breathing: Thoughts are taken up more deeply.

Warming: A deep, affectionately warm enthusiasm can be developed for the world and the spiritual essence behind it (for instance, in philosophy, art, religion).

Nourishing: Thoughts are less superficial and are taken at a deeper level ('digested'). A deeper understanding of the world, life and people comes about.

Secreting: A new understanding emerges as to what is essential and inessential. Everyday events become less interesting (fluid thinking), whereas greater insights arise concerning the 'big questions of life' (crystalline thinking).

Maintaining: Greater connections are perceived and the ageing human being gains wider vistas.

Growing: The ageing person develops a rich inner life.

Reproducing: Due to this greater overview, life-experience and understanding of how things are connected, the ageing person can achieve mature creations that are of lasting value. This specially applies to artists.

These processes together bring about the 'wisdom of age.' If these life forces turn mainly to the physical and material body and are not used for spiritual development then disturbances in the body can occur.

The soul life in old age

In the soul feelings can arise such as sadness regarding the loss of beauty and bitterness because of the loss of bodily pleasures. These privations can kindle the wish to make up for these losses by other means. The drive to enhance the intensity of experience can lead to extravagance (for instance, misuse of medicines; enlargement/beautification of living quarters; flashy ornaments/jewellery) or specialists are sought who can free the person from age-related miseries with medicines, treatments or operations.

Deep down, however, the ageing person knows that the ageing process cannot be halted through outer manipulations. The resulting dissatisfaction can be countered if the person manages to loosen the grip of the soul forces on the ageing body. This can be achieved by seeking opportunities that do not stress the fragile body too much, such as contemplative walks, age-appropriate gym and dance, creative and play-like occupations. Apart from these, artistic activities are particularly suited to bring movement and life to the soul through the experience of the rhythm of tension and relaxation. New faculties can develop that will compensate outer loss by inner gains and richness.

In this connection the experience of festivals and celebrations during the course of the year and in one's personal life assume special significance. To this one can add the opportunity to meet socially, to chat and have fun, as well as attending memorial meetings for those who have died, as the soul not only wants to experience joy but also dignified sorrow. 'Taking leave' is in old age a frequent and important experience. It helps ageing people to gradually loosen their earthly attachments and to appreciate that it is the soul and spirit, the immortal parts, that carry and support them.

Total abstinence from all earthly pleasure does not relieve elderly people of dissatisfactions. Making use of still available strengths, accepting their limits, allows the soul to swing between activity and rest and arrive at a peaceful equanimity.

The individuality in old age

For the elderly the radius of action becomes naturally smaller. There are fewer people around who have lived through the same part of history as they have. The few who remain are less mobile and one meets them less often. Friends and relatives increasingly step into the background or die so that there is hardly anybody who knows these old people as they once were. The following generation has other experiences and other outlooks. Developments in the fields of politics and technology, as well as the emergence of different value systems, are not always understandable for an ageing person.

Old age also brings increasing loneliness. The world around them becomes less familiar and considerable effort is needed to understand new developments. Thus the ageing person needs more self-confidence to uphold her individuality and not to lose contact with the world around them. The strength and support needed cannot be drawn from a world they cannot understand. The inner values of religion and philosophy gain in significance. It is at this point that the ageing person can let go of the ties with the material world and instead trust in the life and soul forces. New experiences can then open up and a journey can begin into an unknown and unfamiliar land. This 'journey' is an individual and unpredictable one. The landscapes, paths and the kind of progress made during the journey are determined by one's own life story.

The strength of the 'I' determines how much the 'I' can lead, how lively the journey can be and how manifold the experiences encountered. The surroundings can be either a help or a hindrance. It will depend on the nature of the interaction with the environment whether the spiritual ageing process is experienced as a maturing process or deterioration. Tom Kitwood, the British social psychologist observed, 'Personhood ... the uniqueness of persons ... is a standing or status that is bestowed upon one human being, by others, in the context of relationship and social being.'[1]

Challenging developments in the ageing process

Not all human beings go through the phase of ageing in this (ideal) form, least of all those for whom we offer care. Within our present professional settings we meet two large groupings of people who present us with questions and challenges to our caring capacity. For the sake of clarity they will be described here in terms of their extreme manifestations.

One group comprises those who are confined to bed and require round the clock intensive care. They are never fully awake, have perhaps a stomach-tube and are incontinent. All bodily functions need assistance. They lie in bed for weeks, months, perhaps years without any apparent change in their condition. With good care they do not acquire bedsores or pneumonia or other hardships; they just rest, day-in and day-out until one day, they do become sore or acutely ill and die.

The other group is comprised of those who are generally termed as suffering from *dementia*. They have lost their orientation regarding place (physical world), time (life processes), the situation they are in (soul environment) and their own person ('I'). From an anthroposophical standpoint the use of the term 'dementia' is questionable. Literally translated it means 'without spirit' which negates their being human. Until a more acceptable term is found, it is right to speak of such people as 'people with problems of orientation.'

These people are usually not bedridden; they walk about (often quite a lot) and could in terms of their agility and bodily fitness, easily care for themselves. Because of their lack of orientation, this is not possible. In their feeling-life they show increased sensitivity; this reveals itself in their ability to sense very accurately the mood and attitude of their fellow beings and to react accordingly. As if driven by a hunger for experiences, they are always seeking sensory experiences. They touch, pull, stroke, rock, run, speak — often using stereotypic repetitions and searching for something they are unable to name. Their bearing and behaviour and way of thinking seem to belong to a reality to which 'normal' people have no access. Their speech is often witty and original. Their behaviour can be friendly or aggressive. Expressions of sadness and seemingly unmotivated laughing can suddenly occur. Although their feelings are intense, they do not appear to be conscious.

Changes in configuration

From the aspect of fourfoldness, the characteristics of these two groups point to the different ways in which the configuration of the various parts loosens. In the first group the physical body and etheric body appear to be strongly present. Similar to a sleeping human being, the life processes can continue to work unhindered. These people give the impression of being bodily 'healthy' and those close to them often express pity that they are not able to die. Their state can be compared to a vegetative existence.

The configuration of the human parts is quite different in the second group. Physical body and etheric body which are present retreat in significance. The care for their own body is no longer an issue for these people. The body is rather like a 'vehicle' to transport the soul to experiences. The astral body and the 'I' are intensively and often restlessly occupied with their experiences, albeit with a changed consciousness. They show a loosened configuration and act as if they were independent of each other and can no longer sensibly cooperate.

Soul experience stands very much in the foreground. Traces of a person's individuality turn up in their often bizarre behaviour. It is a mark of their I-quality that they perceive other people's sensitivities when encountering them. One cannot pretend with them as they see through pretence. The connection between their odd behaviour and their own biographies is seen as a starting point in order to understand their current state.

Questions of meaning

Searching for meaning in such destinies, which are on the increase, and seeking an answer is not easy so long as attention is only directed to the outer circumstances. Rudolf Steiner was once approached to give his view regarding a lame and unconscious woman requiring intensive care. Someone suggested that it might be better to allow her to die. Steiner answered, 'No, every day, every hour which she lives on this earth is not only a boon for her but is of meaning to the whole of humanity.'[2] He also commented, 'that the earth has not died already is due to the fact that there are human beings who stay so long in their bodies and thereby transform their body.'[3]

Each day when human beings wake up they lift their body against the force of gravity into an upright position. People confined to bed no longer muster this strength and yet in a subtle manner this force is still at work for it is only in death that the body become entirely subject to gravity. As long as there is still a spark of life in the body, the impetus to uprightness is still at work. This is evidenced by the fact that in spite of years of resting in bed, bedsores do not develop. Only when the life forces are finally in retreat do they occur.

These forces of buoyancy, which from a religious angle may be called resurrection forces, are present in every body so long as there is life. The body, as a part of the earth, is a vessel and expression for spiritual forces. The totality of the life forces in all people, especially those who are severely affected, increases the force of buoyancy against all the depressing, drying-up and hardening tendencies that are present in the world. Such thoughts can motivate the carer and it becomes meaningful when providing good care to a person who seems to be in a vegetative state. It can further motivate the carer to help those who are no longer able to get up to sit at the edge of their bed or to give those who no longer can walk the experience of standing on their own feet, at least once a day. Even the judgement regarding disoriented people that they lead a pitiful and meaningless life and are prey to their own misfortune can be put to one side when spiritual aspects are considered.

If this phase of disorientation is a time of processing their own destiny then every day and hour is of importance for them because it can be a preparation for the time after death. By experiencing this as a reality, which is not our own, they are like a person who looks through a key-hole into new spaces which they will enter when the time arrives. Seen this way, such people are far ahead of us. By encountering them, we can learn that there is more on earth than we can grasp with our reason. In the strange and innocent condition of their soul they demand from us honesty, truthfulness and authenticity.

In view of the increasing number of senior citizens, especially in the industrialized world, the question arises as to whether old age is seen as a burden or whether its hidden meaning may provide mankind with an opportunity to develop faculties which run counter to much of the social coldness, destructiveness and violence of contemporary society.

FURTHER READING

Glas, Norbert, *The Fulfillment of Old Age.*
Kitwood, Tom, *Dementia Reconsidered: The Person Comes First (Rethinking Ageing).*

7. Health and Illness

Health

When seeking the meaning of the word 'health' we find it is related to wholeness. Essentially it is the ability to live in harmony with the surroundings yet separately; the ability to set oneself apart without isolating oneself; opening oneself up but without dissolving.

According to the WHO, health refers to bodily, spiritual and social well-being. It is not a fixed state but is the result of a constant effort to achieve harmony. The leading thought for the following enquiry is not pathogenesis, which relates to factors causing illness, but to the idea of *salutogenesis,* which looks for the forces that maintain or restore health.

Bodily well-being

Bodily well-being, according to *salutogenesis,* denotes the ability of the organism to react sensibly and adequately to the continuously changing conditions and influences to which a human being is exposed (that is, adaptation). According to the salutogenetic model, the healthy organism is not formed by homeostasis but 'by continuous heterostatic processes transforming into homeostatic ones and therefore possessing a high degree of ability for processing and adaptation.'[1] From this point of view, people with a disability or chronic illness can, through the use of specially designed apparatus (for instance, prosthetic aids), cope with their situation and arrange matters in such a way that it leads to a healthy life.

Social well-being

According to the concept of salutogenesis, a healthy soul life is necessary for a sense of social well-being. Healthy soul life is expressed in terms of coherence: a 'feeling of being at one with all there is.' People experience themselves appreciated by society. This applies particularly in the extreme situations of great happiness and deep sorrow. Sharing one's joys strengthens the life forces. When one is in trouble it helps to know that there are people who know and understand you. This gives the strength to endure the worst situations even though the people concerned may not be in your immediate vicinity. But it is not just a question of receiving help from others as offering help to others is equally important for this strengthens the health of one's soul. It is a basic human need to be of social significance for others.

Spiritual well-being

Salutogenesis as far as spiritual well-being is concerned is the ability to be resilient, to possess the strength to withstand attacks of negative, destructive and hostile influences that can depress one and cause illness, even if one is not the target. Speaking of the health of the soul, attention should be directed to personal sorrow. On the spiritual level we experience powerlessness when we are confronted by violence, brutality and catastrophes and are unable to grasp their meaning and do anything about them. Resilience is the strength that allows us not to break down but to develop trust in the meaningful evolution of humankind and to discover the sense and purpose in one's own life. People who are spiritually healthy will be able to see their destiny, whatever it is, in a wider context; they can accept and deal with it because they are able to take a position which gives them the confidence to open up perspectives for the future.

Disturbances in the health of body, soul and spirit

Bodily illness

Symptoms of illness, before they become pathological, are healthy capacities, (for instance, secretion, production of warmth, sensitivity, hardening or dissolving of tissues, tensing and relaxing etc). These processes are only considered illnesses when they occur in the wrong place, at the wrong time and in the wrong intensity. Once they become too strong or too weak and this process has started, it cannot easily be halted.

Whether we are dealing with defence reactions, hyper- or sub-functions, insufficiency, cramps, paralysis, tumours or other failing functions, we need to find the healthy middle position between:

too much — too little
too firm — too slack
too hard — too soft
too tense — too flaccid
too dry — too wet
too pale — too red, etc.

The extremes which appear as illness, in anthroposophical medicine are called cold and warm illnesses. The group of cold illnesses comprises all those that tend towards denseness, blockages and finally lead to a breakdown of substances: hardening, cramp-conditions, stones, and degenerative illnesses. The warm illnesses include those in the direction of fever, hypersecretion, loosening, swelling (for instance, inflammation and allergies). In the warm illnesses the loosening processes are too strong; they are similar to healthy metabolic processes. In the cold illnesses it is the form-giving tendencies that dominate; they have some affinity to those forces that normally belong to the sensory nerve system.

Generally one can observe that illnesses in the first half of life are more likely to be of an inflammatory nature and go in the direction of loosening, whereas in old age the degenerative, hardening tendencies are at work. This may look quite differently when examining individual destinies as illnesses also have a biographical significance. It is not just a matter that one experiences similar illnesses in a different way at different stages in one's life. One needs to consider each case individually.

Soul-related illness

Also on the level of the soul, the balance can become disturbed and feelings of coherence lost. It is in the nature of the soul to live in polarities. There are an infinite number of ways of expressing the ecstasy of joy and the doldrums of despair. In social life we swing between the need to be alone and the need to be with others. We call a person 'well-balanced' who can find the middle between extremes, who can quite happily be on their own and also be sociable in the company of others.

In psychiatric terms there is a disturbance of equilibrium that leads the person in one direction or another or where there is a rapid alternation between extremes making therapeutic intervention necessary. Sometimes this condition may necessitate isolation in order to protect the affected people from themselves or to protect others.

As far as the daily care is concerned a systematic discussion of psychiatric illnesses is not directly relevant. More important is the necessity to draw attention to the phenomena we have to deal with in psychiatrically changed human beings. Basically they show similar tendencies as are shown in bodily illnesses: on the one hand a process of hardening: anxieties, depressions, compulsions, self-destructive tendencies and on the other hand the process of loosening: states of delusion, hallucination and loss of limits. In a manic depressive illness these two states fluctuate which can lead to mania — a heightened sense of well-being. This presents a challenge to our notion of health as being a state of 'well-being.'

Spiritual illness

A basic thought in anthroposophical medicine is that the spirit itself cannot become ill. Therefore we do not speak of 'spiritual disability' but rather impairment of a healthy spirit. A disturbed configuration of body and soul hinders the sound spirit from finding healthy expression. We can perhaps better understand this through an image. If an instrument is faulty even the best musician will not be able play on it to the best of his abilities. If the tools are defective, even the most skilful craftsman cannot produce a masterpiece.

The spirit is fundamentally healthy and is the source that activates all self-healing powers. All therapies work in partnership with this spirit. The following example of the craftsman shows us something else. Functions, which are disturbed by illness or deficiency, can be compared to a range of carving tools, some of which have been damaged or lost. The wood-carver who stands for the spirit can nevertheless successfully ply his craft even with knives that have been hardly used. With perseverance he may be able to achieve the same kind of result that he would have achieved with a full set of tools leaving the lay person unaware of the fact that anything was lacking. This is the principle of rehabilitation.

He can also have his tools repaired or replaced by others because he knows what is missing. This would be healing. In the last resort he might come to the conclusion that he is no longer able to work in this workshop; just as in death the spirit leaves the body without dying itself.

Illness and destiny

Illnesses are a part of a life story. Every illness makes that clear. Some things must change. The causes of many illnesses can be found in the past, for example, in one's life style or nutritional or environmental factors which have led to a disturbance, deficiencies or damage. The organism demands an appropriate compensation and a change in life circumstances.

The question of what has caused an illness remains open. If the past does not provide us with clues for understanding what is happening, then attention must focus on the future. When one looks with the help of the healthy spirit, for a wider context and recognizes the illness as a challenge by destiny then it is necessary to question its meaning. What does this illness mean for me? Can I learn from it? Where does it come from? Where will it lead?

To achieve that delicate balance of achieving health is a dynamic process. Any disturbance challenges the organism to regain its balance. According to Glöckler, the point is not to avoid causes of ill health but to wrestle with them and to strengthen oneself in the process. In so doing, it is necessary to recognize one's own limits in coping with stress and, if possible, to strengthen one's capacity to cope. The effort to re-establish the balance requires a process of learning new faculties. If that can be achieved, the outcome in the end may be a correction and/or an enrichment that strengthens the self-healing powers.

While care in itself cannot heal, it can create the conditions for healing to take place. On a bodily level, care can support the life forces; on a soul level, care can bring about helpful encounters which will strengthen the balance of soul and the feeling of coherence; on the spiritual level, care can recognize unique individuality and help an old person to find and walk the path which seems in harmony with what destiny wants.

FURTHER READING

Bentheim, Tineke van, *Home Nursing for Carers.*
Bie, Guus van der and Machteld Huber (Eds.) *Foundations of Anthroposophical Medicine: a Training Manual.*
Bott, Victor, *An Introduction to Anthroposophical Medicine.*

Evans, Michael and Ian Rodger, *Healing for Body, Soul and Spirit: an Introduction to Anthroposophical Medicine,* (in America: *Complete Healing*).

Glöckler, Michaela, *Salutogenesis: wo liegen die Quellen leiblicher, seelischer und geistiger Gesundheit?*

Glöckler, Michaela, *Medicine at the Threshold of a New Consciousness.*

Zieve, Robert, *Healthy Medicine: A Guide to the Emergence of Sensible, Comprehensive Care.*

8. Repeated Earth Lives

Anthroposophy regards man as a reincarnating being. The 'I,' the individual core of the human being, comes to the earth in order to have experiences and take responsibility for them. With death life has not finished, rather a new form of existence begins in which the 'I' processes and evaluates the experiences of the past life and integrates them. Life on earth can in this sense be seen as a day in school, with other days to follow. The aim of repeated earth-lives is that individuals, step by step, can perfect themselves until they have reached the next stage of development.

From this point of view 'blows of destiny,' such as 'misfortune,' 'illness' or 'bad luck' in a single life should not be understood as mere accidents. They should be seen rather as important life experiences that serve to gain new forces, capabilities and recognitions. They are the consequences of a chain of causes, as well as a preparation to acquire new faculties for new tasks, which perhaps arise only in later incarnations.

Life after death

The physical body is the bearer of the other human parts. The body belongs to the earth and is prepared by the mother from the time of conception. Step by step the higher human parts incarnate, until by the middle of life they are closely linked together and connected to the earth. Thereafter begins the gradual loosening of the human parts (excarnation).

This loosening results in a drying up of the physical body because the life-processes exert ever less influence. Instead the energy of the life-processes can be used for enhancing consciousness. The loosening of the astral body from the physical is seen in the fact that physical structures lose their former shape (for instance, formation of wrinkles; diminished muscle tone). The structuring forces of the astral body now become available for the life of the soul. All these processes are experienced as an ageing of the body. At the same time, they allow for a freer unfolding of thinking and the soul-life. The 'I' takes on the task of holding together and ordering the thinking and the soul-life and developing it further.

Dying is that phase of life when the 'I,' the astral body (soul) and etheric body (life processes) begin clearly to separate from the physical. Death occurs when this separation is completed and the higher parts 'cross' the threshold.

The physical body after death

Immediately after death, of the four human parts of the human being, the physical body is the first to disintegrate. This is given back to the earth as dead matter at the funeral. The other three parts are still interconnected in the immediate surroundings of the earth, freed from the physical body.

The etheric body after death

The state of loosening immediately after death permits the 'I' to perceive an image of what has been imprinted on the life body (etheric body) during the course of life. People who have had a near-death experience describe this life-tableau as a big panorama with all the images side by side.[1] It is significant that neither the soul nor the 'I' have any influence on them. The panorama is simply there to be seen.

This stage lasts for about three days. During this time the life body (etheric body) gradually dissolves into the etheric mantle surrounding the earth. The life-tableau becomes weaker until it vanishes.

Abilities and habits, which a person has gained during life (for instance, cycling; singing; thinking; playing; making music) and which have become patterns imprinted on the etheric body, dissolve into the earth ether, from which the etheric body originated.

The astral body after death

The astral body (that is, sensations, feelings, consciousness) and the 'I' are now in the astral world which is the home of the astral body. In this sphere the astral body and the 'I' experience a retrospective view, showing the events the soul has undergone in the past life, not as a tableau but as experiences, starting from the last moments before death and moving backwards. Now it is not their *own* feelings that are experienced but the feelings that these individuals have caused in their social contacts during life on earth. One now experiences every joy or pain that one has caused to others. This can be called the complementary experience of one's own deeds. Here it is a matter of undergoing this process without the possibility of making any changes. And yet, a deeper insight into social living is engendered.

The soul-forces which the 'I' could not control during life (for instance, greed for food; addiction to drugs; uncontrolled drives) demand their tribute. The longing may still be present but there is no material body to allow satisfaction. Accordingly, these unsatisfied desires cause distress. This period of life between death and new birth lasts approximately one third of one's past life and corresponds to the time the person has spent sleeping. In religious tradition this time is called purgatory, in esoteric traditions purification or kamaloka. Only when the soul has fully freed itself from 'lusts and attachments' is it ready to loosen itself from its configuration and become one with the astral world. Nevertheless there are remnants (for instance, unresolved relationships, unsolved problems) of the soul-forces left behind in the astral world.

The 'I' after death

Now the 'I' widens itself into the next sphere which is the homeland of all humankind and the individual core of being. In religious terms it is the realm of the Creator, of God. Here a meeting takes place with one's higher 'I' which means that part of the 'I' that up until then has not been able to fully incarnate on earth. What remains from the past earth-life are those faculties that the 'I' has achieved during life on earth (for instance, patience; attention; empathy; musicality; ability to love). The results of living on earth enrich and perfect the higher 'I.' In so doing the human being encounters the 'Judge.' The spiritual powers that created him evaluate and put into order these newly achieved faculties. In that process some gaps may become evident which need to be considered in the future development. In this way the impulse for a next incarnation and its tasks comes about. A 'draft plan' is made from the viewpoint of the spiritual world. However not all details of the future life are determined. The 'plan' draws attention to the fact that particular faculties need to be developed, supplemented or enhanced in order to resolve earthly entanglements and to fashion new relationships.

Preparation for a new incarnation

Most of the time and effort is devoted to working out the 'plan' for the shaping of the new physical body. Enriched and stimulated by the impulses of this 'plan,' the 'I' now seeks responsibility for the process of self development. To this end, a new life on earth is required. Only then can a confrontation take place that allows the process of individual development. The human being, restricted by the limitations of a physical body, is nevertheless independent in his consciousness. This means liberated from the effects of cosmic influences and the 'I' is forced into making decisions and taking responsibility for them. Therein lies human freedom to choose, to err, to correct and to take responsibility.

The path towards the earth

When the 'I' sets out in the direction of the earth, the path leads again into the astral world where the soul composition is newly arranged to form the new astral body. The residue that was left behind has now been integrated into the astral body. The 'I' now attaches itself more strongly to the astral body and both draw closer to the earth and 'look out' for the chance of a physical incarnation which is suitable for what its soul and spirit require. That these early delicate contacts can be made is for instance confirmed by women who soon after conception feel that contact has been made with them at the time of conception which gives them the certain feeling that pregnancy has started. The conception initiates a new incarnation; a new life begins. The value of knowing about reincarnation lies in the recognition that human beings, as they appear on earth, are not the product of chance. Every incarnation is the result of a long development with all its attendant problems and errors but equally with all the gifts and chances. The recognition of reincarnation and karma allows us to have a broader understanding of how the human being and nature (etheric world) are related to the social environment (soul life) and other human beings.

FURTHER READING

Achiati, Pietro, *Reincarnation in Modern Life.*
Bauer, Dietrich, *Children who Communicate before they are Born: Conversations with Unborn Souls.*
Fallaci, Oriana, *Letters to a Child Never Born.*
Steiner, Rudolf, *Reincarnation and Karma.*
—, *The Meaning of Life.*
—, *A Western Approach to Reincarnation and Karma.*

9. The Concept of Care

Care takes place at the levels of the body, of inter-soul connections and of spiritual understanding.

For the *body* it is important that the organism finds its own balance amidst the continuously changing states of the body. In order to support this process the carers attend to the body, observe the seven life processes (that is, breathing; warming; nourishing; secreting; maintaining; growing; reproducing) and by so doing support and regulate the influences on these life-processes.

On the *soul level* health is supported and fostered by carers making the surroundings comprehensible and suitable for an older person through offering stimulation and giving orientation. By relating to the carer, the older person experiences clarity and dignity which facilitates a sense of coping with circumstances and the possibility of identifying with oneself and the environment and giving a sense of coherence.

On the *spiritual level* care focuses on trying to give to the elderly person confidence in her own destiny (karma); to facilitate an awareness that one's life is of significance and is linked to all humanity and the earth. The carers act supportively when they show respect for the whole and healthy individuality of people entrusted to them. They enter into the care relationship authentically with honesty, love for and interest in the older person.

As far as bodily care of the patient is concerned, carers need to pay daily attention to the bodily functions, supplemented, where necessary, by preventive measures, physical practices and medical prescriptions. For instance, knowing of, and being able to apply, rhythmical massage according to Wegman-Hauschka and basic sensory stimulation can enhance the care for the body. All these have a harmonizing effect that go beyond daily hygiene. On the soul level, touch, which is part of the daily care for the body, can be transformed so that it is like a conversation.

Attention should also be paid to ensuring that speech, expression and gesture are congruent with content, that one always remains courteous and has in mind the basic rules governing social interaction. The surroundings of the bed, ward and treatment room should be furnished in such a way that it stimulates the soul. Carers should also pay attention to their own appearance. Orientation for patients can be facilitated by a clear daily timetable and by keeping appointments that have been made. Elderly people should also be encouraged to have opportunities to express their own opinions.

The spiritual effectiveness of care comes about when carers can see themselves and the patients from a different perspective. This implies taking seriously the fact that every human being (including the carer) possesses a healthy spiritual core regardless of how they might appear (old, ill, disoriented etc.) and despite limited possibilities to express themselves through body and soul. To believe that truth, beauty and goodness live in every human being is a pre-requisite for holding this attitude. Knowledge of the transcendental nature of man and belief in reincarnation may help in developing this trust.

Professionalism in care is founded on the acquisition of knowledge and through practice and reflection. Professionalism enables carers to prepare for their task, plan their daily work, execute their plans and afterwards to reflect upon them. Besides professionalism every carer brings their own biography with its strengths and weaknesses. All of this is brought to bear in order to support the elderly person and to accompany them on their way. Carers can also take on a mediating role by asking other people for help and by promoting contact with relatives, doctors, therapists, friends and others. However, carers cannot be expected to identify totally with the older person.

Older people bring with them their own biographies. Their particular needs are the reason for the caring interaction. That caring interaction is both the basis and centre of the relationship between patient and carer. These needs may constantly change depending on the effectiveness of care. Beyond this, the encounter between patient and carer can intensify inasmuch as the experiences gained in this interaction can be integrated in one's own biography. In so doing, the caring action assumes values that go beyond the duty of care. Through the effort to integrate these experiences at all levels into one's own life, a positive gain is achieved for all. With every caring interaction a chance is offered that through it something totally new or never before imagined can develop.

Care becomes a path that can be integrated into one's own biography. This path can lead either to recovery, to integration of illness and impairment, or it can lead towards acknowledging one's own process of dying. The concepts of fourfoldness, threefoldness and of the senses, are conceptual models drawn from Rudolf Steiner's anthroposophy that support and facilitate carers in sensing and recognizing the spiritual core of every human being.

FURTHER READING

Benner, Patricia, *From Novice to Expert: Excellence and Power in Clinical Nursing Practice.*
— **(Ed.),** *Interpretative Phenomenology: Embodiment, Caring and Ethics in Health and Illness.*
Buber, Martin, *I and Thou.*
Löser, Angela Paula, *Pflegekonzepte nach Monika Krohwinkel.*

PART 3

Guidelines for the Application of the Anthroposophical Model of Care

10. Application of the Model of Care to Practice

As was mentioned in the introduction, the model of care should not be seen in isolation as another model, but be seen as a development of care models. In this chapter there is a scheme showing aspects from four-foldness and the theory of the senses as well as individual, biographical aspects. These may help planning, putting into practice and documenting a care plan.

The system devised by Monika Krohwinkel is provided as an example, as this is the system currently most in use. The questions formulated will help provide a checklist based on an anthroposophically image of the human being. This model of care will help inspecting authorities to recognize the specifically anthroposophical elements which inform our care institutions.

Who is the 'resident'?

The concept of 'resident' is used here for the elderly living in a care home. We have used 'she' simply because the majority of these residents are female. In general terms, the method is applicable to both women and men.

10.1 Ability to communicate

Fourfoldness

Physical level
- Is the resident able to communicate verbally?
- Is she able to communicate non-verbally (that is, through the use of sign language, shaking head, eyes, mime, gesture)?
- Is she in need of aids (for instance, glasses, hearing aid, symbol chart, PC, special telephone with large/programmed digits, special call-sound)?

Level of life-processes
- Are there illnesses that impair or limit communication (for instance, Parkinson's disease, depression, dementia)?
- Does she use breathing patterns to communicate?
- Do the carers, or does the resident know, when she needs the toilet? (See also 10.6 *Ability to urinate and defecate.*)
- How does she express her sense of well-being or ill health or pain?

Level of soul
- How does she communicate her feelings?
- Does she need special objects to help (for instance, a favoured blanket, photos, soft toys, etc.)?
- Does she express her feelings in a particular way (for instance, a cry of excitement, some verbal formulation, kissing)?
- Does she engage in social activities (for instance, hairdresser, games, study, prayer, conversation groups etc.)?
- Which language or dialect is her mother tongue?
- Does she express herself in pictures?
- Does she use stereotypical phrases (for instance, Where is my mother)?
- Does she create her own words?
- Does she mix her words when expressing herself?
- Is she interested in media (for instance, books, news, journals, radio, TV, internet, telephone)? (See also 10.9 *Ability to occupy oneself.*)

Individual level
- How conscious is she of herself?
- What image does she have of herself?
- With whom does she have any personal connection?
- Does she speak to others or to herself?
- Can she take in communication and understand it?
- What kind of communication does she prefer?

Aspects from the theory of senses

Sense of touch
- Communication by touch (for instance, rubbing in of oil, basal stimulation).
- Self-stimulation where there is lack of communication (for instance, rubbing, scratching, masturbation).

Sense of life
- The manner of communication can indicate bodily condition:
  — logorrhea (that is, excessive use of words);
  — elective mutism (that is, the condition of being unwilling to speak as a result of a physical or psychological disorder); and
  — speech in symbols.

Sense of own movement
- Outer movements and thought movements are connected.
- Understanding connections.
- Showing skills.
- Gesture or mime used for communication.

Sense of balance
- Ability to concentrate, to stick to one topic without losing the thread.
- To relate things to oneself or to one's surrounding (for instance, to say 'one says' or 'one does' instead of 'I say' or 'I do').
- To have her own opinion.

Sense of smell
- Smell as a source of information.

Sense of taste
- Tasteful manner of expressing oneself.
- Choice of words (for instance, flowery, polite, factual, nasty).

Sense of sight
- Ways of seeing and viewing; considerations for the future.

Sense of warmth
- Ability to communicate warm-heartedly to others; temperament heated by discussion; anger, cold shoulder, cynicism

Sense of hearing
- Ability to listen, be inwardly still, to hold oneself back.
- Ability to be open.

Sense of language
- Sensory or motor speech impairment.
- Speaking in images or through actions.

Sense of thought
- Understanding the 'message,' realizing what is meant.
- Recognizing the background or reasons for something.
- Unable to understand and do what is asked.
- Agnosia (that is, loss of the ability to interpret sensory stimuli, such as sounds and images).
- Apraxia (that is, total or partial loss of the ability to perform coordinated movements or manipulate objects in the absence of motor or sensory impairment).

Sense of self and others
- Having connections with others.
- Maintaining relationships.
- Understanding others.
- Ability to put herself in someone else's shoes.

Biographical aspects

- How does the resident wish to be addressed?
- Are there other residents who might have something in common with her (for instance, origin, language, profession, interests, date of birth, experiences)?
- Is there anything in the care facility that might have some biographical significance for the resident (for instance, kitchen, library, music room, stables)?

10.2 Ability to move

Fourfoldness

Physical level
- How agile is her physical body?
- Is she able to walk, stand, get up, sit on the edge of her bed, in bed or on a chair?
- Can she turn around, change her position?
- Are the joints flexible?
- What prevents free movement?
- Are there bodily deformities?
- What does she need to move freely?
  — firm shoes,
  — walking stick,
  — glasses,
  — hearing aid, etc.
- Is she in need of other aids?
  — personal help for walking.
  — zimmer frame.
  — wheelchair.
  — mechanical aids to get up, etc.
- Are her surroundings wheelchair friendly?
- What other facilities are available?
  — unobstructed corridors, passageways,
  — hand-rails or other safeguards,
  — non-slip floors,
  — notice boards for directions,
  — safe steps,
  — locked/unlocked doors,
  — sufficient and adequate spaces for people to freely move around,
- Is the bed restrictive in any way?
  — can she get into and out of bed?
  — is the bed convertible?
  — can she use the bed handles?
  — what harnesses are required/available?
  — is a bed guard needed?

- Is it necessary to apply movement exercises (for instance, Bobath or other kinesthetic exercises)?

Level of life-processes
— are there any illnesses that hinder movement?
— are they connected with spasticity, lameness or sensory disturbances?
— is a tremor evident?
- Is there any impairment of gross or fine motor movement?
- Does the resident suffer from dizziness? (See also 10.3 *Ability to maintain vital functions of life.*)
- Are the medicines used helpful or do they cause impairments?
- Does movement positively or negatively influence digestion?
- Does the resident take walks after meals? (See also 10.6 *Ability to urinate and defecate.*)
- Does movement influence breathing, positively or negatively?
- Do breathing problems require a particular position?
— are muscles involved in breathing able to function correctly? (See also 10.3 *Ability to maintain vital functions of life.*)

Level of soul
- Does the resident enjoy moving or is stimulation necessary?
- Is she restricted through her emotional state (for instance, tendency towards depression)?
- Is she interested in recreational provision made for residents (for instance, festivals, excursions, holidays)? (See also 10.9 *Ability to occupy oneself,* and 10.12 *Ability to secure and shape social relationships.*)
- What currently occupies the resident emotionally? (See also 10.13 *Ability to deal with existential experience of life.*)

Individual level
- At which stage is the resident in her development?
- What needs to happen for something to move, loosen, renew?
- What things stir the resident personally?
- Does she show interest in biographical work?

Aspects from the theory of senses

Sense of touch
  • Frequent touching supports identification with one's own body.

Sense of life
  • The urge to move is a manifestation of life.
  • Inability to move demonstrates:
    — a feeling of stagnation,
    — a feeling of imprisonment,
    — a feeling of being stuck.
  • Utterances of moodiness and discontent are connected with this
    sense.

Sense of own movement
  • Interrelation between self-movement and experience of gravity.
  • Lack of self-movement can lead to urge to set the environment
    into movement.
  • Certain stereotypic movements transmit a specific body-con-
    sciousness.

Sense of balance
  • This sense atrophies if a person does not move.
  • Can lead to emotional disturbance (for instance, 'Help, help, I'm
    falling!').
  • Lack of inner balance can lead to giving up (for instance, 'You
    do it nurse, you can do it better').

Sense of smell
  • Good or bad smells can motivate movement.

Sense of taste
  • Lack of movement reduces appetite.

Sense of sight
  • For someone who cannot move, the experience of movement can
    nevertheless be gained by following the movements of objects
    with the eyes:
    — trees in the wind,

— small animals,
— a mobile,
— carers walking to and fro,
— the view of a busy road, park.

Sense of warmth
- Movement produces warmth.
- Warmth (also warmth of soul) makes movement possible.
- Cold stiffens movement.

Sense of hearing
- By the tone of the voice soul-movements can be recognized.
- Sound can stimulate movement (for instance, dancing).

Sense of language
- People with limited movements are often reduced to gestures and mime thus lessening the ability to express oneself. This may give a misleading impression of disinterest.

Sense of thought
- Mobility of outer body and thought are connected.

Sense of self and others
- Mobility allows a person to express herself in manifold ways.
- Loss of mobility can lead to social isolation.

Biographical aspects

- Biographical development is a movement.
- In which direction does the person move (that is, path of life, conduct of life)?
- What role did movement play in her past life (for instance, sport, dancing, travelling, rambling, physical work)?

10.3 Ability to maintain the vital functions of life

Fourfoldness

Physical level
- What size and what weight is the resident?
  — overweight?
  — underweight?
- Is the physical body intact or are parts missing (for instance, amputations, breast removal, organ removal)?
- Is the resident dialysis-dependent?
- Are prostheses or substitute medicaments used?
- Is the skin healthy (that is, evidence of bedsores, cuts, fungal infection, dandruff, ulcers)?
- At which places are respiration rate, pulse and temperature measured?
- What kind of environment is required?
  — room temperature
  — humidity
  — ventilation
- Which medicines are in use?

Level of life-processes
- *Breathing*
  — How is her breathing?
  — Does she suffer from irregularities and under what circumstances (for instance, infections, cough, blockages, mucus, vomiting)?
  — Are the causes known?
  — Does she need particular supports (for instance, bedding, external stimulation, exercises, medicines, oxygen)?
- *Warming*
  — What is her body temperature?
  — Does the resident feel cold or perspire easily?
  — Does her temperature regime need special support (for instance, bath supplements, sources of warmth)? (See also 10.7 *Ability to dress,* and 10.4 *Ability to care for oneself.*)
  — How is the circulation (for instance, cold feet, cold hands, blue lips)?

• *Nourishing*
  — What is her nutritional state?
  — What sort of appetite does she have?
  — How is her metabolism (that is, constipation/diarrhoea)?
  — Are the causes known?
  — What kind of support does she require?
  — Are metabolic illnesses known (for instance, diabetes mellitus)?
  — Has she been given any prescriptions? (See also 10.5 *Ability to eat and drink.*)

• *Secreting*
  — How much does she drink?
  — Does she tend to dehydrate? How does this show itself?
  — Does she retain liquids? Where are the deposits?
  — Is there a need for nocturnal urination?
  (See also 10.6 *Ability to urinate and excrete* and 10.5 *Ability to eat and drink.*)

• *Maintaining*
  — What is the state of the skin?
  — Where there are wounds, what is their appearance?
  — Are the causes known?
  — What prescriptions are given?
  — How well do wounds heal?
  — What factors influence healing?
  — Are there any deformities resulting from rheumatism or arthritis?
  — Where prostheses are used: how are they maintained?

• *Growing*
  — Are there any outer or inner tumours (for instance, boils, old age patches, warts, birth-marks)?
  — Are they being treated and how?
  — Are they regularly checked and recorded?
  — Are there irregularities in hair and/or nail growth?
  — Does the resident need to gain or lose weight?
  (See also 10.5 *Ability to eat and drink.*)

• *Reproducing*
  — Has the resident given birth?
  — Are there any peculiarities in the reproductive organs (for instance, prolapse of womb, prostate enlargement)?
  (See also 10.10 *Ability to feel and conduct oneself*)

Level of soul

• What measures does the resident take to maintain her health?
• What habits and rituals does the resident follow to maintain her health?
• What is the relationship of the resident to her state of health?
• How does this show (for instance, complaining, being negative, being over-demanding on herself)?
• Are there certain states of her soul that are influencing her vitality (for instance, joy, excitement, anxiety, sorrow)?
• Are there any forms of stimulation that could positively influence her vitality (for instance, singing, visits, media, participating in events)? (See also 10.9 *Ability to occupy oneself.*)
• Does she have a zest for life?
• What is she averse to?
• Is she in pain?
• How doe she cope?
• Can she keep to prescriptions? (for instance, diets, exercises)

Individual level

• How does the resident consider her state of health?
• How competent is the resident in administering her medicines?
(See also 10.11 *Ability to live untroubled in secure and stimulating environment.*)
• Is she fond of life?
• Would she like to die? (What makes her hold on to life?)

Aspects from the theory of senses

Sense of touch

• Consciousness of her own body (including prostheses and other gadgets).
• Ability to set her own boundaries.

Sense of life
- Feeling of well-being.
- Ability to notice the following functions and point them out (for instance, hunger, thirst, need to get fresh air, need to use toilet.

Sense of own movement
- Mobility, flexibility, initiative, motivation.

Sense of balance
- Standing in the midst of life, keeping a sense of balance, taking herself seriously and keeping within bounds.

Sense of smell
- Acceptance (sympathy/antipathy).
- Smells which are indicative of specific illnesses (for instance, acetone).

Sense of taste
- Appetite.
- Having a taste for life.

Sense of sight
- Views on own state of health.
- Perspective.

Sense of warmth
- Ability to be aware of her own state of warmth and to react appropriately.
- Ability to be enthusiastic.

Sense of hearing
- Listen to what her body is saying.
- Openness to suggestions regarding health.

Sense of language
- What is our state of health telling us?

Sense of thought
- Questions about the senses.
- The meaning of life and the value of health.

Sense of self and others
- Loneliness — integration.

Biographical aspects

- Are there moments or specific occurrences that are known to have affected the resident's present state of health (for instance, accident, illness, trauma, abuse of drugs or alcohol, medicines, hard labour, war, a prolonged stay in the tropics, hereditary influences)?
- Do memories exist that directly influence her state of health:
  — breathing (for instance, to become calmer, to create anxiety)
  — warming (for instance, cold winters long ago, hardships, my loving mother)
  — nourishing (for instance, memories of favourite dishes)
  — secreting/reproducing (for instance, taboos related to culture or education: a woman not wanting a male carer, shame at being constipated).
- What attitude does the resident have towards her own biography?
  — having had a fulfilled life?
  — what is still possible?
  — what hopes does she have?

10.4 Ability to care for oneself

Fourfoldness

Physical level
- Is the resident in a position to care for herself? (See also 10.2 *Ability to move.*)
- What does she consider most important for her bodily care?
- What utensils are required (for instance, comb, brush, nail-set, toothbrush, razor, etc.)?
- What gadgets are required (for instance, handles, seating)?
- Are they available and usable and are they clean?

Level of life-processes
- What are the habits for body care (for instance, special times and frequencies for showers, baths, foot-baths)?
- What is the condition of skin and hair (for instance, dry, scaly, greasy)?
- What is done for these conditions?
- Are there any allergies or inflammations?
- What are the causes?
- What should the carer remember in daily contact with the resident?
- How does the resident cope with caring for her finger/toe nails?
- How does she cope with her hair care?
- Does she visit the hairdresser, chiropodist?
- How does the resident cope with her dental care?
- Are there any wounds, swellings or lacerations?
- Where are they located and in what condition are they?
Are there prescriptions for these conditions? (See also 10.3 *Ability to maintain vital functions of life.*)
- What cosmetics does she like?
- Does she need treatment with ointments/oils?
- Does she need rhythmical massage?

Level of the soul
- Does she pay attention to self-care?
- What sequence of self-care does she want?
- Which habits and rituals does she favour?

- What water temperature does she prefer?
- What hairstyle does she prefer?
- What perfumes does she prefer?
- Are cosmetics used?
- Does she want to use make-up?
- Are there any preferences with respect to bath essences (for instance, stimulating or calming)?
- Do cultural or religious rituals have any significance for her? If so, which ones?

Individual level
- Is the resident conscious of her body/body-care?
- Is it possible through bodily care to support consciousness (for instance rhythmical oiling, ablutions etc.)?
- Can her consciousness of self be influenced by body-care?
- Does she use a mirror?
- How does the resident cope with exposure of private parts?
- Does the resident have a preference for a female or male carer?

Aspects from the theory of senses

Sense of touch
- The quality of touch (soft, rubbing, scratching) and reactions to it.
- Self-awareness — awareness of body boundaries.
- Distance and proximity.
- Body care as help for incarnation/excarnation.

Sense of life
- Stimulation, refreshment, calming.
- Feeling well.
- Over-demanding, exhaustion.

Sense of own movement
- Self-perception in movement.
- Body-care as movement exercise.

Sense of balance
- Experience of own body centre, of own body space.

• Experience of space (important for bedridden and immobile patients).

Sense of smell
• Fragrances stimulate sense of well-being.
• Sympathy — antipathy.

Sense of taste
• Encounters are conducted with dignity and taste.

Sense of sight
• Sight protection (sunglasses).

Sense of warmth
• Room- and water temperature.
• Avoid chilling.
• The warmth organism can be stimulated.

Sense of hearing
• Adequate decibels.

Sense of language
• Idiom.
• Way of conversing.

Sense of thought
• To include the resident.
• To inform the resident.
• Washing shows respect for the resident.

Sense of self and others
• Care is encounter with the other.

Biographical aspects

• Are there any memories of experiences, conditions, education, cultural backdrops which relate to body care or influence it (for instance, 'My mother handled me so roughly', 'My husband likes ...')?

- Ritual religious ablutions.
- Traumatic experiences (for instance, abuse, rape and guilt can be connected to the urge to have 'to wash something away').
- Are there old habits of life (for instance, to have a bath once a week).

10.5 Ability to eat and drink

Fourfoldness

Physical level
- Are the teeth in good order?
- Are the false teeth in order and fit well?
- Can something be improved?
- Has the food to be mashed?
- Who is the dentist? When was the last appointment?
- Can she eat normally at the table?
- Are special eating utensils required? (for instance, plate, cutlery, anti-slip mats)
- What drinking utensil is required?
- Is serviette protection needed?
- Is help needed to get eating started?
- Is the skin of the mouth healthy?
- Can she swallow normally?
- Can the resident coordinate chewing, swallowing and breathing? Are there any dangers?
- Is motor activity of mouth disturbed (for instance, drooling)?
- Is tube-feeding necessary and are all utensils and food for this available?
- What is the body-weight and size?
- How good is the appetite?
- What is the frequency and times for the meals?
- Does the resident have any particular eating habits?
- Is a special diet required?
- Is additional food required between mealtimes?
- Is there a heightened need of calories in evidence?
- What is the speed of eating (that is, fast/slow)?
- Does the food have to be kept warm?
- Are there any illnesses in the mouth or digestive tract?
- How good is the flow of saliva?
- Are there any allergies?
- Is the resident inclined to nausea, vomiting or diarrhoea?

Level of life-processes
  • What is the nature of the drinking habits (for instance, amount drunk, ability to drink independently)?

Level of soul
  • What preferences does the resident have regarding eating and drinking?
    — Is sweet or savoury food preferred?
    — Can she taste the food?
    — Are there items she rejects?
    — Where does the resident prefer to eat (that is, alone or in dining room)?
    — Has she any preferences as to where she sits at the table?
    — Does she appreciate the culture of communal eating?
    — Does she choose food at the table by herself?
    — Does she dress specially for mealtimes?
  • Is the resident able to cut and spread butter/margarine on her own?
    — What support does she require?
    — Can she feed herself?
  • If a tube is in place can additional food be given orally?
  • What preparation of food is preferred (for instance, vegetarian)?
  • Are there any religious/cultural taboos relating to eating and drinking?
  • Are there any personal rituals (for instance, saying grace, reading newspaper at breakfast table, having a glass of wine, having coffee when getting up, eating out once a month)?

Individual level
  • What value does the resident attach to eating and drinking?

Aspects from the theory of senses

Sense of touch
  • Consistency of food presents different touch experiences.
  • By eating and drinking a part of the outer world becomes part of the inner world.

Sense of life
- Communicates feeling of hunger, feeling of being satisfied.
- Feeling well as a result of eating.
- Eating gives comfort.

Sense of own movement
- Movements, such as cutting, spreading, etc.
- Chewing movement, tongue movement.

Sense of balance
- Right amounts distributed in a balanced way throughout the day.

Sense of smell
- Fragrance of food enhances appetite.

Sense of taste
- Is enhanced by spices, salt, herbs, sugar, honey or combinations.

Sense of sight
- Enjoys pleasing appearance of food
- Enjoys tasteful table decoration, colours, etc.
- Appropriate clothing.

Sense of warmth
- Room temperature.
- Temperature of meals and drinks.

Sense of hearing
- Decibels in surroundings, sounds and noises (for instance, radio, rattle of china, other disturbances).

Sense of language
- Conversational speech.
- Way of speaking.

Sense of thought
- Saying grace.
- Conversations during meal.

Sense of self and others
- The table community.
- Dignified mood at mealtime.
- Do carers join in the meal?

Biographical aspects

- People connect certain foods with certain events. This should be respected in large kitchens (for instance, seasonal festivals, Sundays, birthdays).
- Social background also plays a role.
- Introduce new menus with care and allow time to try out.
- Elderly people love old habits as they provide security.
- The constitution of elderly people is not always able to cope with big changes (for instance, from meat eating to vegetarian, the length of the intestines is not sufficient).
- Habits, like a glass of wine at table should not be frowned upon; the decision to change or to hold on to what one was used to should rest with the elderly person.

10.6 Ability to urinate and defecate

Fourfoldness

Physical level
- Is the resident continent?
- Is she able to use the toilet independently?
- Does she need special equipment?
  - Moist cloths
  - Special toilet paper, etc.
- Can the resident assume the right position?
  - If not, what are the difficulties?
  - How can the problem be solved? (See also: *Ability to move*)
- What aids are required?
  - Hand bracket
  - Heightening of seat
  - Footstool, etc.
- If toilet cannot be used, what alternatives are required?
  - Toilet commode
  - Bed pan
  - Urinal
  - Female urinal, etc.
- Can resident use aids herself; what support is needed?
- Is there any incontinence?
  - What materials are required?
  - Product, size, quantity
- Is a condom-urinal in use?
- Does the resident use a permanent catheter?
  - Can she handle it?
  - Is the required material at hand?
  - Is the address of the specialist available?
- What other excretions are in evidence (for instance, sweat, sputum, tears, wound-secretion). (See also 10.3 *Ability to sustain vital functions of life.*)

Level of life-processes
- What are the defecation habits of the resident?
  - Frequency, timing, quantity, consistency
- Are laxatives required?

- Does she require a special diet in this respect?
- What urine excretion habits has the resident?
  — Frequency, quantity, appearance/odour, nocturnal urination
     (frequency, causes)
- Is bladder/toilet training pursued?
- Is a urinary control protocol carried out?
- At what times and how often is the incontinence protection (for
   instance, pads) changed?
- Does the resident take sufficient liquids? Is a record kept? (See
   also 10.5 *Ability to eat and drink.*)
- Has the resident an oedema?
- Does the resident use diuretics?
- Does the resident perspire excessively? Are the causes
   known (for instance, use of deodorant or astringent bath
   supplements)? (See also 10.4 *Ability to care for oneself.*)
- What quantity of sputum is produced? If exceptional, are the
   causes known?
- How are the ears, nose and navel cared for?
- What considerations are given to secretions from wounds?

Level of the soul
- Does the resident know when she needs the toilet and does she
   communicate this?
- Does she suffer pain?
- What would be helpful to her at the toilet (i.e, newspaper)?
- In the case of incontinence, how does she cope?
- Are problems of excretion caused by the mental state?
- Does the resident exhibit any idiosyncrasies? If so, what?
- How can these be creatively tackled?
- Where can complaints be lodged? (And will they be heard?)

Individual level
- Is there privacy in place for toilet purposes? (See also 10.10
   Ability to feel and conduct oneself as a man or woman.)

Aspects from the theory of senses

Sense of touch
- Sensing the skin in relation to secretions and excretions.

• Part of the inner world is passed to the outside world.

Sense of life
• Sense of well-being can be influenced by the process of excretion.
• Change in moods through these processes (for instance, through constipation/blockages).

Sense of own movement
• Outer movement enhances digestive and excretion processes.

Sense of balance
• Drawing attention to oneself by certain behaviour relating to excretion.

Sense of smell
• Smells are a way of providing information about contents of excreted matter.

Sense of taste
• Taste provides information about structure and chemical composition.
• The laboratory replaces the sense of taste in determining nature of content.
• Tasteful treatment in dealing with excreted matter.

Sense of sight
• Colour, form, quantity, appearance.
• Sight protection.

Sense of warmth
• Room and body temperature and excretion (for instance, cold inhibits process of excretion).

Sense of hearing
• Sound of excretion is embarrassing to most people.

Sense of language
• Certain body-language can indicate need for use of toilet.

Sense of thought
- Processes concerned with excretion can preoccupy the mind.
- Lavatorial language. Events connected to process of excretion are often used to express certain thoughts or feelings.

Sense of self and others
- Is there any danger in seeking to reduce the resident's focus on excretion?

Biographical aspects

- The faculty of excretion is learned as a child and then executed independently throughout life. For an adult person having to depend on the help of others in this private sphere can have a severe impact.
- The act of excretion is usually conditioned by socio-cultural influences. Elderly people bring with them habits and sensitivities.
- The older person might have experienced being excluded — 'excreted' in the social realm (for instance, when someone is shunned in a group or dismissed from a team or separated from the family).
- A biography resembles the process of digestion: learning, producing and passing on relate to accepting food, digesting and excreting it.
- Blockages such as constipation and diarrhoea can be a response to coercion.
- Excretion can be linked to the temperaments (for instance, melancholics — constipation, sanguines — diarrhoea).
- This can be balanced by providing adequately adapted food.
- What did this person do before she was unable to go to the toilet?
- Does this person want to 'get rid of something' (for instance, feeling of guilt, doing away with old habits)?
- Or does the person want to 'hold on to something' (for instance, convictions, habits, objects)?
- Is this person ready to depart from life? What is still holding her back?

10.7 Ability to dress

Fourfoldness

Physical level
- What kind of clothing does the resident wear?
- Does the resident have adequate footwear of the right size?
- Does she have adequate clothing for different conditions?
  - — For the wheel chair
  - — Easy to fasten
  - — Easy to dress and undress
  - — For special occasions
  - — Non restricting
- How is the clothing cared for and by whom?
- Where is it stored?
- Is it marked by name?
- Which nightdress is worn/needed?
- Can she handle her clothing herself?
- What help does she require?

Level of life-processes
- Is the clothing suitable to support the temperature regime?
- Do certain body areas need special attention (for instance, feet, legs, bladder/kidneys, shoulders, pulse)?
- Is the head sufficiently protected against cold and outer influences through wearing a hat, nightcap or sun hat? A cold head could be a reason for sleeping problems.
- Are there allergies and/or skin irritations/sweat irritations which are reactions to certain fabrics?

Level of soul
- What is the preferred clothing of the resident?
- Does she prefer a particular style?
- Does she differentiate between weekdays and Sundays/festive days?
- What does she not like to wear?
- What does she prefer to wear when sitting in the wheelchair, armchair or bed?
- Does her clothing support her personality (for instance, elegant,

sporty, practical)?
- Does clothing serve as a status symbol (for instance, a suit, an apron, a professional outfit)?
- Does she like to wear jewellery, shawls and ties?
- What does she want to express (for instance, joy in life, memories, status)?
- Which colours, patterns and fabrics does she prefer?
- Does she make any special demands (for instance, in relation to hairstyling)?

Individual level
- Is there a connection between self-esteem and the clothing chosen?
- Does her present appearance match her level of self-esteem?

Aspects from the theory of senses

Sense of touch
- Suppleness, quality of fabric: rubbing, scratching, soft, silken ...
- Separation of the inner from the outer world.

Sense of life
- Feeling secure and well through possessing good clothing.

Sense of own movement
- Well-fitting clothing enhances movement.
- Safe footwear prevents accidents.

Sense of balance
- Identification with one's clothing.

Sense of smell
- Clean and cared-for clothing.

Sense of taste
- Tasteful clothing for the person and the occasion.

Sense of sight
- Pleasant appearance: 'Don't I look pretty?'

• Beauty strengthens the will.

Sense of warmth
  • Clothing fit for the climate.
  • Sense of warmth and production of warmth are reduced in old
    age.

Sense of hearing
  • No prejudices in respect to clothing.

Sense of language
  • Clothing as means of expression: colour, shabby, stylish.

Sense of thought
  • 'Do clothes create people?'

Sense of self and others
  • Clothing is a cover, what (who) is hidden within?

Biographical aspects

• People connect clothing with certain events (for instance, confir-
  mation, first homemade dress, wedding dress).
• Clothing is also part of the socialization process. A classical
  example can be found in Rilke's life, where his mother had
  wished for a daughter and dressed her son in girl's dresses.
• Buying clothes can be an expression of the state of soul (for
  instance, to enhance feeling of security, to conform to a social
  group).
• Memories of crisis situations can lead to habits of clothing (for
  instance, to go to bed fully dressed with shoes on ...).

10.8 Ability to rest, relax and sleep

Fourfoldness

Physical level
- Where does the resident sleep best?
- Structuring the bed environment:
  — where is the bed positioned?
  — at which side is the wall?
  — at which side does she get out?
  — how is the room lit?
  — what is the room temperature?
  — does she like the window open/closed?
- What is the usual position for falling asleep?
- How should the bed be arranged?
  — mattress
  — pillows (for instance, hard, soft, number, size)
  — blanket/duvet (for instance, feather, wool, synthetic)
  — provision of support cushions
- What does the resident require in bed (for instance, night dress, head cover, bed socks)? (See also 10.7 *Ability to dress.*)
- Which items does she require on the bedside table?
  — clock
  — telephone
  — lamp
  — photos
  — paper tissues

Level of life-processes
- What are her sleeping habits?
  — length?
  — time periods?
  — sleeping pattern?
  — midday rest?
- Does she feel hunger/thirst at night?
- Does sleep bring relaxation?
  — If not: have the causes been investigated?
- Are there any sleep interruptions? If so, what are they caused by?
  — sounds

— light
— digestive problems
— neighbour
— night staff

- Does she have to visit the toilet?
- Has she to be bedded at night? (See also 10.2 *Ability to move.*)
- Does she take sleeping pills?

Level of soul
- Are there certain rituals before going to sleep, in the morning, after rest hour?
- Does she dream much?
- How is her state of soul when awake at night?
- How is the breathing during sleep (that is, breathing is an expression of tension and relaxation)?
- Does the resident have fears of darkness and noise?

Individual level
- Can she go to sleep with a sense of trust?
- What might help her (for instance, prayer, poetry, conversation, first appearance of the night staff, knowing who is around)?
- Does she have an urge to speak to the night staff about her worries, problems, anxieties, happy events, and memories?

Aspects from the theory of senses

Sense of touch
- How strongly is she incarnated?
- Can she let go?

Sense of life
- Feeling unwell, anxiety disturbs sleep.
- To have a sense for how much sleep is needed.

Sense of own movement
- Wishes, worries and conscience can make a person restless, disturb sleep and cause sleeplessness.
- In which direction does life move?

Sense of balance
- A balanced human being sleeps well.
- How is balance and orientation achieved during the night?

Sense of smell
- Familiar smells give reassurance.
- Waking up as a result of strange smells.

Sense of taste
- Order in the room.
- 'When everything goes according to my wishes I can sleep well.'

Sense of sight
- Light conditions influence sleep:
  — brightness of night lights
  — which light is used by the night staff?
  — stand-by lights of electrical appliances can disturb sleep.

Sense of warmth
- Sleep is dependent on the right temperature
- Balanced temperature for the whole body (that is, feet, legs, hands, head, back).
- Bed temperature.
- Room temperature.
- Warmth of soul.

Sense of hearing
- Noises impact on sleep and relaxation.
  — positive: familiar sounds, music
  — negative: sudden noises, din.

Sense of language
- The way of speaking.
- Communication brings security and promotes sleep (for instance, a few words, signals, signs, bell).

Sense of thought
- Thoughts are different during night.
- The faculty to concentrate is different.

• Lack of clarity, bad thoughts disturb sleep.

Sense of self and others
• The knowledge that there is someone who knows me and cares for me gives confidence and promotes sleep.

Biographical aspects

• What did the resident do before admission when unable to go to sleep?
• Are there still memories which impact on sleep (for instance, times of war)?
• Does she have anxieties or non-resolved experiences?
• What are feelings about dying (for instance, 'Sleep is the little brother of death')?
• About one third of life is spent sleeping. What a person experiences during sleep and how much that person is refreshed, influence the relation to sleep and everything connected to it.

10.9 Ability to occupy oneself

Fourfoldness

Physical level
- Is the resident able to occupy herself independently?
- What sort of help is required to achieve independence? (See also 10.2 *Ability to move,* and 10.3 *Ability to maintain vital functions of life.)*
- What is the course of a typical day? What are her wishes to improve it?

Level of life-processes
- What stamina does she have to engage in an occupation? (See also 10.3 *Ability to maintain vital functions of life.)*
- How often can she pursue an occupation? (per day, per week ...)
- How does occupation improve health?

Level of the soul
- How much is she motivated to occupy herself?
- What are her interests?
- What programmes in the media attract her? (See also 10.1 *Ability to communicate.)*
- What are her sources of information?
  — About her close surroundings (for instance, staff, co-residents)?
  — About in-house events (for instance, newsletter)?
  — About personal contacts (for instance, visits, telephone)?
  — About local and world events? (for instance, newspaper, TV)?

- Is the resident inclined to physical activity?
  — taking care of own body care
  — caring for her room/flat
  — contributing to domestic tasks
  — participating in handwork, crafts
  — engaging in physiotherapy, ergotherapy (that is, treatment of disease by muscular exercise)
  — gym

— going for walks, hiking
— swimming

• Does she like artistic activities, for instance
    — painting
    — modelling
    — singing
    — dancing, eurythmy

• Which events is she interested in?
    — social events
    — festivals
    — film shows
    — slide shows and lectures
    — theatre
    — concerts
    — courses (for instance, calligraphy, biographical work, memory training)
    — working groups
    — conversation groups
    — religious events
    — further education

• Does she enjoy games? Which ones?
• Does she have a sense of humour?
• What does she not like?
• Does she prefer to do activities in groups or by herself?

Individual level
• Which activities are a clear expression of her individuality?
• Which activities could be offered her that would therapeutically support and strengthen her personality?

Aspects from the theory of senses

Sense of touch
• Differentiated activities offer manifold contacts with the world and give opportunities to meet oneself in various ways.

Sense of life
  • Meaningful occupation increases contentment and joy in life.

Sense of own movement
  • Every kind of occupation facilitates movement experiences and furthers outer and inner mobility.

Sense of balance
  • A balanced relationship between activity and rest.

Sense of smell
  • What is right for one person is not necessarily right for the other.

Sense of taste
  • To find the appropriate thing for each one.

Sense of sight
  • Activity provides a different outlook on life.

Sense of warmth
  • To warm towards something and to become enthusiastic increases one's quality of life.

Sense of hearing
  • To occupy oneself with something can provide an opportunity for developing new ideas.

Sense of language
  • Occupation as a means of expression.

Sense of thought
  • Activity stimulates thought.

Sense of self and others
  • Activity provides opportunities for encounters in a variety of ways.

Biographical aspects

- What used to be her main interests?
- How did she used to organize her day?
- What pleased her especially?
- By understanding the soul-spiritual nature of the human being, one can see activity to be more than just following one's
  whims.
- As a being conscious of her self, a person has the inclination to
  become active in and with the world, thereby to develop and
  meet questions of life.
- One can distinguish three basic activities. During the different
  periods of life, the emphasis changes:

  1. To get to know (absorbing phase), childhood and youth: to
     get to know the world, to adapt oneself and inform oneself
  2. To stand up for oneself (productive phase), middle section of
     life: to conquer one's place in the world, to hold on through
     work and the founding of a family
  3. To reflect (contemplative phase), old age: to digest the experi-
     ences of life, to integrate and transform.

10.10 Ability to feel and conduct oneself as a man or woman

Fourfoldness

Physical level
- Does being a man or a woman find expression in:
  — appearance?
  — bodily constitution?
  — clothing?
  — laundry?
  — perfume?
  — cosmetics?
  — shaping one's surroundings?

Level of life-processes
- Are there changes through hormones in the male/female character?
- Are there gender-specific illnesses (for instance, enlargement of prostate, prolapse of womb)?
- Are there any gender specific cancers?
- Are there any sexual diseases?

Level of the soul
- How does she feel about herself as woman?
- How does she feel when in the company of women/men?
- How does she react to female and male carers?
- Are there gender specific occupations or activities in which she/he would like to engage (for instance, cooking, tea-parties, hobbies, needlework, pub going)?
- Is there sexual desire? (Is there privacy?)
- Does she feel sexually harassed?
- What arrangements are there for proximity to or distance from the other sex?
- Is her privacy respected?
- How does she deal with feelings of shame and disgust?

Individual level
- How does she cope with the role of woman?
- How does she think of herself as a mother?

• Does she have a life partner?

Aspects from the theory of senses

Sense of touch
  • Touching another body.
  • Arousal through touching of erogenous areas.
  • Closeness/distance

Sense of life
  • Feeling well in one's own body
  • Hormonal effects/changes.

Sense of own movement
  • Movement patterns can be female or male in character.

Sense of balance
  • Being in accord with one's own gender.

Sense of smell
  • Female/male odours.
  • Perfumes as aphrodisiacs.

Sense of taste
  • Tasteful conduct with the other sex.
  • Experiencing the other sex as complementary to one's own.

Sense of sight
  • Beauty, attraction.

Sense of warmth
  • Interest.
  • Openness to others.
  • Excitability.
  • Search for adequate contact.

Sense of hearing
  • Being able to hear the human essentials beyond gender specific roles.

Sense of language
- To understand sex specific utterances as a wish to communicate.

Sense of thought
> Procreation is a creative act between two human beings. The exchange of thoughts is also a creative act.
> — positive: fruitful conversation
> — negative: ambiguous talk.

Sense of self and others
- The core of the human being is not determined by sex.

Biographical aspects

- Did women/men play a particular role in her life (for instance, mother, father, siblings, daughters, sons, teachers, employers)?
- Was it possible to live as woman or was this suppressed?
- Was she a mother, if so, where are the children now?
- Are there any sex-specific burdening events? Do resentments persist?
- Did they have a 'gender-specific profession' (for instance, midwife, soldier)? Has this profession shaped them?
- Do they have any gender-specific ideals, norms, and anxieties?
- Did they possess gender-specific pride (for instance, 'I was the village beauty', 'I could beat any man!' 'I have always honoured women')?

10.11 Ability to live untroubled in a secure and stimulating environment

Fourfoldness

Physical level
- What conditions are necessary for her to feel secure in her environment?
- Prevention of falling
  — safe footwear
  — spectacles, hearing aid
  — handrails
  — non-slip surfaces
  — help-call system
  — other aids (see also 10.2 *Ability to move,* and 10.7 *Ability to dress.*)
  — lighting conditions
  — accident prevention measures
- Is the resident oriented to her immediate surroundings?
- What spatial/local gadgets are required to assist orientation?
- Are there any steps, lifts, balconies, open windows and exits that might be dangerous?

Level of life-processes
- Is the resident in a position to explore her environment?
- Are there environmental factors detrimental to or endangering her health (for instance, noise, bad air, moisture, toxic food, unhygienic conditions)?
- Is it necessary to have laboratory checks (for instance, blood-sugar, etc.)?
- How is medical supervision guaranteed?
  How well are dangerous substances controlled (for instance, medicines, cleaning materials)?
- What support does she need?
- Does the resident have a sense of time?
- What aids are required for orientation in time?
- Is adequate nutrition guaranteed? (See also 10.5 *Ability to eat and drink.*)

Level of soul
- Is she aware of her situation?
- What help is needed?
- Is she able to weigh up situations?
- Does she feel secure in her present situation?
- What gives her that feeling of security?
- Does she suffer from anxieties?
- Is there a supporting social network in existence and within reach (for instance, family, friends, neighbours)? (See also 10.1 *Ability to communicate.*)
- Does she suffer from depression?
- Is there any evidence of a suicidal tendency?
- Does the resident endanger herself/others?
- Is the resident able to recognize dangers and avoid them (for instance, lift, stairs, open window)?
- Can she leave her room/house independently and find it again?

Individual level
- Does the resident feel acknowledged and accepted?
- Does she have a sense of identity with her own person and her biography?
- Is she able to deal with her personal affairs?
- Does she have a carer? Has she given power of attorney to someone? Has she made a living will?
- Does she need support? Is support adequately arranged?

Aspects from the theory of senses

Sense of touch
- To embrace, support, hold hands, cover up in bed/chair ...
- Appropriate touching provides security.

Sense of life
- Insecurity weakens the life-forces.

Sense of own movement
- Security promotes ability to move.
- Insecurity impedes.

• Limitations of movement decrease possibilities for information and orientation.

Sense of balance
• Insecurity throws a person out of balance.
• Balance exercises help towards on inner security.
• Prevention of falling.

Sense of smell
• Familiar smells promote security.
• Typical smells help in orientation (for instance, food smells, coffee, soap, smell of Christmas) or give warning (for instance, burning, gas, rotten food).

Sense of taste
• Familiar food gives security (as with mother at home).
• Familiar accustomed surroundings create security and order (an inner order).

Sense of sight
• Clear and visible conditions, order and information bring security.

Sense of warmth
• A warm atmosphere provides relaxation and familiarity (also warm colours, wood, tactile fabrics).
• Coldness indicates rejection.
• Sensitivity for cold and heat warns of dangers (for instance, sunstroke, over-hot water bottle, too lightly dressed in winter).

Sense of hearing
• Familiar sounds transmit security: (for instance, songs from childhood and youth, folk music, classical music).
• High decibels decrease security; friendly background music and quiet sounds remove stress.
• Unfamiliar sounds can cause anxiety.
• Being hard of hearing causes insecurity

Sense of language
  • Hearing one's mother-tongue gives confidence.
  • Clear articulation and speaking slowly increases security.

Sense of thought
  • Clear and understandable information, truthful statements understood, perceived and recognized.

Sense of self and others
  • To be accepted gives a feeling of home.

Biographical aspects

  • Linking up to one's own biography helps a person to feel accepted and 'at home.'
  • This is supported when an old person can live in a place that is near to her own biography or has the possibility of spending time in the kitchen, common room, and tearoom or having familiar objects around her. (See also 10.12 *Ability to secure and shape social relationships.*)
  • Did biographical events occur which led to lasting attitudes, such as mistrust, anxiety, dependency, feeling threatened or persecuted, having a heightened need for reassurance?

10.12 Ability to secure and shape social relationships

Fourfoldness

Physical level
What external preconditions are needed to maintain social connections? (See also 10.1 *Ability to communicate,* 10.2 *Ability to move,* and 10.9 *Ability to occupy oneself.*)
- What financial resources are available to maintain social connections?
- Which provisions are available (for instance, transport)?
- Does she receive regular newspapers, journals and other literature?

Level of life-processes
- Where and how did she live before becoming dependent on help?
What were her usual pursuits (for instance, walking in the park, shopping, sweeping the courtyard, walking the dog, visiting the cemetery, going to the cinema on Mondays)?

Level of soul
- What is her ethnic and cultural origin?
- Does she belong to a community of faith?
- Does she belong to a particular professional association, club, interest group, self-help group?
- What were her contacts before becoming dependent (for instance, relatives, friends, neighbours)?
- What connections does she want to maintain?
- What new contacts could possibly be offered?

Individual level
- Who are her closest contacts?
- Which of the carers feels specially responsible for her?

Aspects from the theory of senses

Sense of touch
- To feel at one with oneself without losing touch with one's surroundings.

- Carefully assess what kind of needs exist in order to cultivate social contacts.
- What are her wishes?
  What does she not want?

Sense of life
- To perceive where and with whom she feels at ease.

Sense of own movement
- 'To move towards each other.'

Sense of balance
- Right measure of distance and closeness.
- The need of the person to be alone or together with others and to make such provision.

Sense of smell
- Sympathy and antipathy.

Sense of taste
- Who fits together, what fits together?

Sense of sight
- What perspectives arise from these relationships?
- How does one perceive oneself in relationships?

Sense of warmth
- Loving attention.
- Commitment.

Sense of hearing
- Belonging.

Sense of language
- Speaking the same language.

Sense of thought
- Exchange of thoughts.
- Common views, individual views.

Sense of self and others
- Perceiving and recognizing others.
- Experiencing community (common ideas) with others.
- Inner safety.

Biographical aspects

Is there a wish to straighten out stressful relationships?

Knowledge and appreciation of the biography can give hints on how to support the creation of social relationships.

People who no longer live in their own home country can suffer from feelings of homelessness. It is not always helpful to try to imitate their cultural customs (for instance, food that is not quite like the native one). Pictures and ethnic music and conversation might be of benefit.

Decreasing short-term memory can give way to childhood and youth memories (for instance, longing for mother). Even well integrated elderly people can be overcome by home-sickness. This pain is quite legitimate. It can be alleviated for a time but can never be removed. Taking it seriously helps.

10.13 Ability to deal with existential experiences in life

Characteristics of existential experiences

Our path in life is shaped by events and experiences that can either support or endanger us. All of the life-activities dealt with so far can be existential experiences. The remarks regarding 'individuality' and 'biography' have pointed to this. Existential experiences are those experiences that touch us in our innermost being, when they confirm our existence or (perhaps more often) when they threaten us.

The joy in a success, overcoming an obstacle, resolving a problem, surviving a danger, solving one of life's riddles are as much existential experiences as suffering from conflict, grief, loss of a loved human being, anger regarding suffered injustice, disappointment concerning a failed action, remorse for a mistake made or shock of sudden bad news.

The central existential experience is the awareness of the finality of our earthly life. Nothing touches our existence so inevitably as the certainty that we have to die one day. Nothing awaits us with more certainty than our own death. It invites us to confront our own existence and poses the question whether there is a continuation of this existence after death. This question stands, more or less consciously, in the background of all our life-experiences and fashions our image of world and man.

Elisabeth Kübler-Ross described the stages passed through by a human being on her way towards death.[1] She blazed a trail for a differentiated understanding of the process of dying and showed that dying begins not shortly before death but gradually develops in five stages:

- denial
- anger
- bargaining
- depression
- acceptance

The same phases are also relevant for other existential experiences. When caring for and accompanying elderly people, they can help us to interpret and understand reactions and give us beacons in our own caring endeavours.

Dependency as an existential experience

Acknowledgement of the need for help has a severe impact on the biography of an older person. It signals the exit from life and leads with certainty, though perhaps with detours, towards death. In the process of coming to terms with this, human beings go through similar phases as in dying. They will not necessarily follow the same sequence and not always arrive at the same result. Often the character of one phase becomes the pattern of reaction over a longer period of time. It is important to be sensitive to such reactions and ways of behaving. Once this basic tendency is recognized, a focused approach is possible.

Denial

For some elderly people care is understood as a service that you can 'buy' in order to continue life as usual. Not infrequently they have their own ideas and wishes regarding this service. We should value these considerations, ideas and wishes, recognize them positively as signs of their own activity, to which we should respond as far as possible.

Anger

Some people react with anger to the fact that they are in need of help. They experience their restricted independence as a loss and accept caring actions with some reluctance. Carers should not take this reaction personally. Anger frequently covers up deep feelings of disappointment, anxiety and embarrassment.

Apart from having conversations with the resident, the carer needs to develop a sensitive approach in order to transform the energy of anger into an ability to help oneself and to mobilize this energy into self competence. In time, self-care, such as getting up oneself and the using of aids can be practised.

Bargaining

Dissatisfied with their situation, some people seek ways of not being dependent on help. They consider their condition to be temporary one.

- The doctor made a mistake and their condition is not really bad.
- Young people talk so indistinctly that she cannot hear what they say.
- The bed is placed in the wrong place and therefore she cannot sleep well.

- Some may hide their dirty laundry so that no one can see that
  they are incontinent.
- They stay in bed in order that no one can see that they cannot
  walk any more.
- If only they were given the right medicine they would be all
  right.

In some ways these people know that they can no longer manage by themselves, however they cannot accept that fact and try to delay the inevitable. It is of little benefit if carers get themselves involved in such discussions. It is more important to show one's readiness to help but in an unobtrusive manner. It may also be important to point out certain professional information regarding the value of the care that is being offered.

The key concept is trust. When a human being does not feel overpowered by care and rather sees it as something offered, it will be easier to accept the new situation. The expectation that help *has* to be accepted is as much an abuse of power as a refusal by carers to perform necessary professional tasks.

Depression

Some people react with resignation at having to become dependent on help ('It's of no use, I'm worthless.'). Resignation is a heavy burden on the resident and also saps the strength of the carer. Resigned people need us to understand their state. Indicating that they are still capable of doing all kinds of things usually makes them more despondent because it does not match with reality. Through an understanding and accepting attitude, the carer can try to find out whether the resignation originates from disappointment ('I have worked all my life for myself and now I have to finish in such a way') or if she feels lonely ('No one is there for me any more'). Warmth of soul shown through interest and patience can create an atmosphere where biographical conversations become possible. It may be necessary to engage professional help, perhaps pastoral assistance, in order to motivate the person to take life into her own hands again.

Taking part in the social life of an institution for the care of the elderly, with common meal times, encounters and events can kindle new motivation. It is not infrequent that people meet with others who are in the same situation, through sharing conversations they arrive at positive solutions. Occasionally even new friendships develop which help over-come the sense of loneliness and open up perspectives for the future.

Acceptance

The willingness to accept a new life-situation and assistance is rarely present at the beginning. Acceptance should not be mistaken as a sign of giving up ('Just go ahead, you can do it better than I, you know what is right.'). Even in a state of dependency, the 'I' is always a factor which should be reckoned with. Acceptance is an achievement in terms of existential experience. To accept a state of dependency is the basis of a caring partnership in which the resources of the person needing care are of equal value to the abilities of the carer. Care in this sense becomes a real encounter and a gain for both parties.

Stages of confronting existential experiences

The phases described by Kübler-Ross are not only applicable to exis-tential experiences such as dying or becoming dependent on help, but to other events where an intensive confrontation with the personality takes place. The dynamics of the process of transformation can be expressed in five stages.

1. Bewilderment

A typical reaction to the profound experiences, noted in Kübler-Ross' phase of denial, is astonishment irrespective of whether it stems from a great joy, sorrow or shock (that is, 'that's unbelievable', 'that's beyond my grasp'). This impression has first to be processed before one can actually realize it.

2. Working through

Confronting the facts is the first step in processing. The stronger the person is touched the livelier this process is. Comparable to this phase is the process in dying described as anger. In the warmth of engagement the 'I' becomes manifest. I am challenged but I don't give up.

3. Transformation

The third phase, which Kübler-Ross has called 'bargaining,' shows itself in the effort to integrate existential experience into one's life. Incisive experiences show that life cannot continue as before. The new situation demands a change in the old behaviour pattern. Holding on to what one is accustomed to and familiar with is a natural reaction. 'Perhaps it is possible after all to continue with life as it was before, perhaps I have to adjust here or there to some degree but on the whole I can carry on without a big change.' The realization that looking for quick compromises does not provide an answer for the future leads to the fourth phase.

4. Pausing

This phase is comparable to what Kübler-Ross has called 'Depression.' There is a general sense of helplessness. Nothing works anymore. Perhaps during a short moment of contemplation it becomes clear that things cannot go on as they used to do. In the stillness of this pause lies the chance to let go of the accustomed and to experience something new. The strength arising from such a moment of quiet can only be noticed when for at least some of the time, all activity ceases. In this listening phase a new impulse for action can be perceived.

5. Agreement

In agreement the changed life-situation integrates the person once again into the wider context. She is able to identify and affirm her new existence. What is new is accepted and a new and changed life begins.

Existential experiences are experiences of the self

We have described existential experiences as experiences which touch individuals to the very core of their being. It is not a matter of checking that all stages take place according the above sequence. Time is needed in order to accept them and integrate them into one's own life. This process and the stages through which it passes bear the signature of the 'I.' It is only in this way that the 'I' can adapt to the new and absorb it. By accepting such an experience as a challenge, the 'I' tries to find the point which lies between total rejection and acceptance without questioning. Whenever anything new arises over the horizon, the 'I' is involved. Everything new is an opportunity to learn, it is a wake-up call for the 'I.' What confounds us most presents the strongest call.

Endnotes

Introduction
1 Meleis, A.I. *Theoretical Nursing, Development and Progress.*
2 Steppe, Hilde, 'Pflegemodelle in der Praxis,' *Die Schwester/Der Pfleger,* 29.291-93, 1990 April.

Chapter 6
1 Kitwood, Tom, *Dementia Reconsidered: The Person comes First (Rethinking Ageing),* pp. 7f.
2 Related by Alexander Strakosch, a teacher of the Waldorf School in Stuttgart.
3 Comment from a letter of Carl Unger.

Chapter 7
1 Glöckler, Michaela, *Salutogenesis: wo liegen die Quellen leiblicher, seelischer und geistiger Gesundheit?*

Chapter 8
1 See Moody, Raymond, *Life after Life,* Bantam Books, and Ritchie, George, *Return from Tomorrow.*

Chapter 10
1 Kübler-Ross, Elisabeth, *On Death and Dying.*

Bibliography

Achiati, Pietro, *Reincarnation in Modern Life,* Temple Lodge Press, Forest Row 1997.
Bauer, Dietrich, *Children who Communicate before they are Born: Conversations with Unborn Souls,* Temple Lodge Press, Forest Row 2005.
Benner, Patricia, *From Novice to Expert: Excellence and Power in Clinical Nursing Practice,* Prentice Hall, New Jersey 2001.
— (Ed.), *Interpretative Phenomenology: Embodiment, Caring and Ethics in Health and Illness,* Sage Publications, California 1994.
Bentheim, Tineke van, *Home Nursing for Carers,* Floris Books, Edinburgh 2006.
Bie, Guus van der and Machteld Huber (Eds.) *Foundations of Anthroposophical Medicine: a Training Manual,* Floris Books, Edinburgh 2003.
Borbély, Alexander, *Secrets of Sleep,* Basic Books 1988.
Bott, Victor, *An Introduction to anthroposophical Medicine,* Rudolf Steiner Press, Forest Row 2004.

Bryant, William, *The Veiled Pulse of Time: an Introduction to Biographical Cycles and Destiny,* Lindisfarne Press, New York 1996.

Buber, Martin, *I and Thou,* Continuum, London 2004.

Burkhard, Gudrun, *Biographical Work: the Anthroposophical Basis,* Floris Books, Edinburgh 2007.

—, *Taking Charge: Your Life Patterns and their Meanings,* Floris Books, Edinburgh 1997.

Camps, Annegret & Ada van der Star, *Menschenkundliche Aspekte zur Qualität in der Krankenpflege,* Urachhaus, Stuttgart 1963.

Evans, Michael and Ian Rodger, *Healing for Body, Soul and Spirit: an Introduction to Anthroposophical Medicine,* Floris Books, Edinburgh 2000 (in America: *Complete Healing,* Steinerbooks, Massachusetts 2005.

Fallaci, Oriana, *Letters to a Child Never Born,* Doubleday, New York 1978.

Glas, Norbert, *The Fulfillment of Old Age,* Anthroposophic Press, New York 1986.

Glöckler, Michaela, *Salutogenesis: wo liegen die Quellen leiblicher, seelischer und geistiger Gesundheit?* Verein für anthroposophisches Heilwesen, Unterlengenhardt 2001.

—, *Medicine at the Threshold of a New Consciousness,* Temple Lodge Press, Forest Row 1997.

Houten, Coenraad van, *Awakening the Will: Principles and Processes in Adult Learning,* Temple Lodge Press, Forest Row 2003.

—, *Practising Destiny: Principles and Processes in Adult Learning,* Temple Lodge Press, Forest Row 2007.

Kitwood, Tom, *Dementia Reconsidered: The Person Comes First (Rethinking Ageing),* Open University Press 1997.

Kübler—Ross, Elisabeth, *On Death and Dying,* Routledge, London 2008.

Lievegoed, Bernard, *Phases: the Spiritual Rhythms of Adult Life,* Sophia Books, Forest Row 1998.

Lievegoed, Bernard, *Man on the Threshold: Challenge of Inner Development,* Hawthorn Press, Stroud 1985.

Löser, Angela Paula, *Pflegekonzepte nach Monika Krohwinkel,* Schlütersche Verlagsdruckerei, Hanover 2003.

Meleis, Afaf Ibrahim *Theoretical Nursing, Development and Progress,* Lippincott Williams & Wilkins, Philadelphia 2006.

Moody, Raymond, *Life after Life,* Rider & Co, London 2001.

O'Neil, George and Gisela, *The Human Life,* Mercury Press, New York 1990.

Ritchie, George, *Return from Tomorrow,* Chosen Books, London 2007.

Soesman, Albert, *Our Twelve Senses: Wellspring of the Soul,* Hawthorn Press, Stroud 2006.

Steiner, Rudolf, *Inner Reading and Inner Hearing,* Steinerbooks, Massachusetts 2008.

—, *The Meaning of Life,* Rudolf Steiner Press, Forest Row 2005.

—, *An Outline of Esoteric Science,* Anthroposophic Press, New York 1997.

—, *Reincarnation and Karma,* Anthroposophic Press, New York 1992.

—, *Theosophy,* Anthroposophic Press, New York 1994.

—, *A Western Approach to Reincarnation and Karma,* Anthroposophic Press, New York 1997.

Treichler, Rudolf, *Soulways: Development, Crises and Illnesses of the Soul,* Hawthorn Press, Stroud 1991.

Zieve, Robert, *Healthy Medicine: A Guide to the Emergence of Sensible, Comprehensive Care,* Bell Pond Books, Massachusetts 2005.